D1590631

Watchful Care

A History of America's Nurse Anesthetists

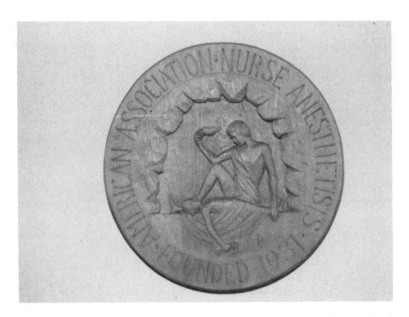

"Watchful Care of the Sleeper by the Light of the Lamp of Learning," the official seal of the American Association of Nurse Anesthetists, adopted in 1940. According to ancient legend, Hypnos, the God of Sleep, daily retired to a ledge in the Cave of Night to seek his rest. To foster sleep and pleasant dreams, he took with him a bunch of poppies that he continued to hold in his hand, even in slumber so profound that his arm slid off the ledge. Morpheus, the versatile God of Dreams, was delegated to watch over Hypnos as he slept, to fend off harm, and to ensure pleasant dreams. In the seal, he is shown holding aloft the Lamp of Learning, by the light of which he keeps his vigil.

The seal was designed by AANA members Louise Schwarting and Lennie B. Dearing, along with W. W. Bowen, MD, and artist Hugh C. Mosher.

Watchful Care

A History of America's Nurse Anesthetists

Marianne Bankert

CONTINUUM · NEW YORK

2004

The Continuum Publishing Group Inc
15 East 26 Street, New York, NY 10010

Printed in the United States of America

Library of Congress Cataloging-in-Publication Data

Bankert, Marianne.
    Watchful care : a history of America's nurse anesthetists /
Marianne Bankert.
        p.   cm.
    Includes bibliographies and index.
    ISBN 0-8264-0510-X
    1. Nurse anesthetists—United States—History.   I. Title.
    [DNLM: 1. Nurse Anesthetists—history—United States.   WY 11 AA1
B218w]
RD80.3.B36   2000
617.9′6—dc20
DNLM/DLC
for Library of Congress   89-9890
                                                                        CIP

To my sister, Nancy

The first few minutes of the flight were smooth and interesting as we flew over lush green jungle. Then the pilot headed for the South China Sea, where we would not be a target for ground fire. . . .

"Would you like to sit up front?" he asked. "I don't have a copilot today. . . . A nurse, huh?" he said, pulling the curtain back across the· door.

"A nurse anesthetist," I corrected. "I put people to sleep for surgery."

"I thought doctors did that."

"They do, but anesthetists do the same thing. Sometimes we work together, sometimes we work alone." He was nodding as if he understood, but I was used to the confusion my job title always produced. "Anesthetists are RNs with two years of additional training in anesthesia," I explained. "Anesthesiologists are physicians."

"And I thought you were a little doughnut dollie," he said with a smile.

—from *Forever Sad the Hearts,* a memoir-novel of Vietnam
by Patricia L. Walsh, CRNA

Contents

Acknowledgments

Nothing is at last sacred
but the integrity of your own mind.

Ralph Waldo Emerson

This study is the result of an invitation by the American Association of Nurse Anesthetists four years ago to prepare a new history of its profession. The last such book, also sponsored by the Association, was Virginia S. Thatcher's *History of Anesthesia, with Emphasis on the Nurse Specialist* (Philadelphia: J. B. Lippincott Company, 1953). It remains a valued resource for much of the profession's early history, a great deal of which would surely have been lost if not for that timely retrieval. While this present study is self-contained, part of it necessarily covers the same ground as Thatcher. In some areas, it has seemed pointless to duplicate entire documents; in these cases I have, in the notes, referred the reader to her study. Yet, even in these matters, the passing of time has provided a broader perspective on the issues and participants. That, combined with subsequent scholarly studies in relevant fields, makes possible a new synthesis.

It is important to note that the AANA, from the beginning of this project, has given me no directions as to how to proceed, what to cover, or what to conclude; nor has it attempted to censor those conclusions. I know that, given the diversity of such a group of practitioners, *all* of whom have passionate feelings about the profession of nurse anesthesia, there is *no* way that this book reflects the perceptions of any particular person, much less the national Association itself. Nor should it be construed as such: I alone am responsible for the views in this study. Some readers will find this attitude of the American Association of Nurse Anesthetists toward a commissioned study either naive, courageous, or confident. I have concluded that it is the latter, and I think the confidence is in the record of nurse anesthetists themselves, and their contribution to the field of anesthesia. To those who disagree with my findings, I urge them to undertake

11

a similar historical journey. I can guarantee that it will be an intellectual adventure.

In fact, it is my hope that the present study will stimulate and
encourage AANA members to continue—or begin—to retrieve the
history of their profession. Perhaps it will be the history of a particular
school or a geographical area; perhaps the history of a significant
individual. Perhaps, also, a greater number of those nurse anesthetists
who have themselves been participants in and witnesses to history-
making events, will be moved to record them. Because the documents
that do exist are so scattered, I have elected to use these pages to
preserve them, making this book, in part, an oral history of the nurse
anesthetist experience. How wonderful it is that people such as Sophie
Gran Winton, Anne Penland, Mary Roche Stevenson, Barbara
Draper, Annie Mealer, Edith Aynes, David Fletcher, and Patricia L.
Walsh have recorded their experiences—painful as they often might
be—and have thus provided us with a glimpse of the wartime anesthetist. How wonderful also that pioneers such as Adeline Curtis and
Gertrude Fife had the foresight to write memoirs; that historian Janet
McMahon interviewed past Association leaders and presidents; that
George Collins, AANA archivist and curator, continues to collect and
display at the national headquarters anesthesia equipment of historic
interest. And what a debt of gratitude is owed John R. Mannix,
former Lakeside Hospital administrator, for urging that Association
proceedings—beginning with the first national meeting in 1933—be
published in a new *Bulletin of the National Association of Nurse Anesthetists*. That published record remains unbroken to this day.

A word must also be said here concerning the contribution of Alice
Magaw. As I advanced in this study, I became more and more convinced that it was not only the achievement of Magaw and her colleagues at Mayo Clinic, but the fact that Magaw documented and
published her work—the earliest paper appearing in 1899—that
nurse anesthetists survived. Early, precedent-setting court decisions
depended not only on expert witnesses and local standards of practice, but cited this undisputed record of accomplishment to support
legally the professional nurse anesthetist. In my own mind it has come
to represent the ultimate example of the axiom, "publish or perish." I
think it not improbable that nurse anesthetists would have fallen
victim to the animus of a small but vocal opposition had it not been for
Magaw's early publications, which gave courts a substantial, scientific
record on which to base decisions favorable to the nurse anesthetist.
(Those familiar with the history of anesthesia know that stranger
things than this have happened in the field: if Crawford Long of
Athens, Georgia, had made public his 1842 work in surgical anesthe-

sia, Morton, Wells, Jackson, and Warren of Boston would not have been variously credited with the anesthesia "breakthrough" of 1846.)

Obviously, I have been aided by many people in many different ways: among them, elected officers of the American Association of Nurse Anesthetists, members of the profession of nurse anesthesia, AANA Executive Staff, anesthesiologists, scholars in the various fields that impinge on this story, librarians, and, of course, there are the essential, supportive friends. It is a pleasure to thank them here, in particular, AANA presidents during the course of this study, CRNAs Barbara V. Adams, Richard G. Ouellette, Peggy L. McFadden, Mary Jeanette Mannino, and Sandra M. Maree; also, CRNAs Dolores E. Biggins, Jan Birnie, Barbara Burner, Ronald F. Caulk, George Collins, Elizabeth Hunt Cote, Aimee Doerr, Patrick M. Downey, Barbara M. Draper, David Ely, David R. Fletcher, Ira P. Gunn, Anita Johnson, Joan Johnson, Robert R. Johnson, Joyce W. Kelly, Ray Luth, Janet McMahon, Janice A. Migon, Thomas E. Obst, Mike Stein, Doris A. Stoll, Edward Thompson, Sandra Tunajek, Patricia L. Walsh, Sophie Gran Winton, Norman R. Wolford, as well as Margaret Faut and Bernadette Roche along with their students at Rush-Presbyterian-St. Luke's and Ravenswood Hospitals, Chicago, respectively. In the Executive Office, I am grateful for the support of John F. Garde, CRNA, Executive Director, Betty Colitti, Jeffery M. Beutler, CRNA, Glen C. Ramsborg, CRNA, Sally Aquino, Karen Farber, the late Lynn Certa, Denise Dungey, Rita Rupp, R.N., and Dorothy Schloderbach.

The cofounders of the Anesthesia History Association, Drs. Selma H. Calmes and Roderick K. Calverley, have been extraordinarily gracious to me. Dr. Calmes shared her studies on women physicians and anesthesiology, and Dr. Calverley—whose historical studies invariably and uniquely include contributions of nurse anesthetists—introduced me to his colleagues, who were most helpful with this project: Drs. George S. Bause, Christopher Lawrence, J. Alfred Lee, and David J. Wilkinson. I am also appreciative of the kindness of Drs. Chang Ho Wee and the late John Adriani.

I am indebted to Major Wynona Bice-Stephens, Army Nurse Corps historian, and Major Susan Steinfeld, as well as to G. Maureen Chaisson-Stewart, George W. Crile, Jr., Audrey B. Davis, Judith DiFilippo, Peter C. English, Debra Hardy-Havens, R.N., Christopher J. Kauffman, John R. Mannix, Doris G. Schreckengaust, Rosemary Stevens, and Lewis E. Weeks; also to librarians/archivists Thomas V. Hull, The American Legion, Andris Kanderovskis and Christa Modschiedler, The John Crerar Library, Eugenia Kucherenko, University Hospitals of Cleveland, Clark W. Nelson, The Mayo Clinic, John Parascandola, National Library of Medicine, Kim S. Perry, The

Knights of Columbus, Joyce Ray, The University of Texas Health Science Center at San Antonio, and Patrick Sim, The Wood Library-Museum. Justus George Lawler, Richard J. Limacher, and Evander Lomke have provided welcome editorial advice, and various kinds of support have come from John Conrow, Gerald Elbin, Seymour Hersh, Louis F. Madda, Frank Madda, M.D., Gloria Marshall, Jo Ann Murray, Isiah Rios, the late Patricia Tervin, and, always, my wonderful family, Nancy and Frank Crotty, Coletta and Michael Neuens, Jean, Marianne, Sharon, Gina, and Jodi.

Introduction
In Search of the Invisible Providers

History is more than a narrative—it is a political stake. . . . History is . . . a place of struggle in itself.

Christine Delphy

The centennial of William T. G. Morton's successful demonstration of surgical anesthesia at Massachusetts General Hospital on October 16, 1946, was marked by the publication of several historical studies. A characteristic of these works was the absence of any substantial and affirmative mention of nurse anesthetists. In part to redress this situation, *The History of Anesthesia With Emphasis on the Nurse Specialist* was published in 1953. In her preface to that book, Virginia S. Thatcher explained, "If the place of the nurse as an anesthetist receives special emphasis in this history, it is because she has been derogated or ignored."

Yet, thirty-five years later, even though they annually administer approximately half of the anesthetics in this country, a national news publication could still headline nurse anesthetists as "the best kept secret in medicine."

As I began this new historical study of the profession of nurse anesthesia, I was, of course, aware of these facts. Yet, like any researcher setting out on the quest for the grail of increased understanding, the discoveries and insights that would occur along this journey could not have been known at the start.

There were surprises.

Surgical anesthesia is a field born in the United States in the mid—nineteenth century, with instant and bitter controversy over rival claimants to its "discovery" (Wells vs. Morton vs. Jackson vs. Long). It is a subject that still stirs passion among devoted partisans. Later in the century, as surgery developed and the need for professional anesthetists became clear, there would arise another controversy—equally long-lived, and often bitter: Who should administer anesthetics?

15

Anesthesia, by that time, *was* recognized as serious business, but one that lacked medical status; it was the surgeon who captained the ship—and collected the large fees. There was no financial incentive for a person holding a medical license to take up the work. Surgeons, in order to advance their specialty, needed reliable, competent, professional anesthetists. They found their answer: nurses. Thus, the first clinical nursing specialty was called into being. And, in its origins, this decision *was* economic—*and* gender-based. It would be decades before the terms "physician" and "nurse" were not synonymous with "male" and "female."

Apart from the few physicians who had a genuine intellectual interest in anesthesia, it would also take years for the economics of anesthesia to make it an attractive area for their colleagues—if at first, only as a supplemental source of income. As this change in attitude developed, it was necessary for physician-anesthetists to establish their "claim" to a field of practice they had earlier rejected. To achieve this end, the accomplishments of nurse anesthetists *had* to be denied or denigrated or ignored.

It was the *process* by which a rival—and less moneyed—group (in this case, nurses) is rendered historically "invisible" that became, for me, the most intriguing part of this study. I frequently felt as though I had been transported to George Orwell's "Ministry of Truth." For example, a myth is launched of the early superiority of British anesthetists—a land, so the story goes, which was never so foolish as to allow nurses to administer anesthetics; the national association of physician-anesthetists backdates its founding to 1905; a new word ("anesthesiologist") is coined in the 1930s to distinguish the work of physician-anesthetists from nurse-anesthetists; "historical" studies are published with titles like *The Genesis of Contemporary Anesthesiology,* as though nothing of significance occurred in the field until the 1920s, when physician-anesthesia began to be effectively organized; and "historical" exhibits and "educational" films are still sponsored that simply ignore the contributions of nurse anesthetists to the field of anesthesia.

It is my hope that the examination of this process in the following pages will be of interest not only to those concerned with the history of anesthesia and nursing as well as the economics/politics of healthcare, but with the history of any group rendered "invisible" (and therefore, powerless) by a denial of its history.

· 1 ·
The Mother of Anesthesia

With Morton's successful public demonstration of anesthesia, one barrier to the development of surgery had been removed. It remained necessary, however, to learn infection control and to develop consistent techniques of anesthesia administration. The understanding and acceptance of antisepsis and asepsis, along with the emergence of the professional nurse, would make possible the continuing advance of surgical science. As Virginia S. Thatcher wryly observed, "To women and to the discovery of 'germs' must go the credit for the greatest contributions to the relief of human suffering during the years between 1860 and 1900." She continued: "To be sure, minute research and improvements in mathematical interpretations of data continued to add to the general body of scientific information, but medical and surgical therapeutics remained static until respectable laywomen invaded the hospital and bacteria were proved to be the specific causes not only of a large group of diseases but also of dreaded surgical infections. Then surgery entered its Golden Age, and the consequences of the indifferent administration of anesthesia were suddenly seen to be important."[1] This "Golden Age" would be embodied notably in the excellence of the Mayo Clinic. It became a mecca for surgeons, and its nurse anesthetist, Alice Magaw, provided such leadership in that new field that her work drew more widespread attention than that of any other member of the Rochester group apart from the Mayo brothers themselves.[2] Magaw would be spoken of by Dr. Charles H. Mayo as "the Mother of Anesthesia."[3]

Germs

A description of surgical practice in the early 1850s has come from Stephen Smith, then junior resident at Bellevue, already an important surgical hospital: "Instruments were placed for ready availability with-

17

out any special cleansing; if dropped during the operation they were used again. The patient was often put on the table unbathed and grimy with dirt; superfluous hair was sometimes shaved off. The only preparation of the surgeon's clothes were measures to keep them from getting soiled. Hands and fingernails were not prepared and assistants came from other ward duties with hands dirtied from multiple sources. Casual onlookers at operations were permitted to introduce unclean fingers into wounds. Sponges were merely washed. Ligatures were left long, one end emerging from the wound."[4] A similar scene at New York Hospital in 1856 was related by Robert Weir, who began there as an assistant to the "junior walker":

> The senior walker was expected to lay out the required instruments, which were stored on a velvet-lined shelf. These he placed on a table and covered with a towel. The sponges, washed out from a previous operation, were kept in a wooden pail of fresh water and were handed to the surgeon during the operation by one of the walkers. "Sometimes" the surgeons and house surgeons washed their hands before operations; however, they did put on clean aprons or gowns, and did not wear, as did many British surgeons, "old coats, stained by the bloody daubs of previous operations." The skin of patients to undergo thigh amputation for compound fracture was washed "with the nice-looking sponges that were filled with disease germs from previous operations which had been quietly multiplying while resting in their pailful of water. Fingers, laden with germs in large quantities on them or under the nails, were stuck into the wounds we made and we further introduced . . . infections and often fatal germs by the brilliant and apparently clean instruments we employed."[5]

Developments in early nineteenth-century bacteriology had revealed the presence of microorganisms or "germs" in organic matter. It was also known that heating killed microorganisms. The explanation for their subsequent reappearance if the substance were allowed to cool came from Louis Pasteur, who demonstrated that this was due to the presence of germs in the dust that settled on the substance. Joseph Lister applied this insight to wound management: since airborne germs caused infection, they should be destroyed on the wound during the operation and prevented from entering it during the healing process. To this end, Lister devised a method for antiseptic surgery, which he announced in 1867. Using carbolic acid as a germ killer, an atomizer was used during the operation to spray carbolic acid solution. The process concluded by using a postoperative system of dressings soaked in antiseptic solutions.

Unfortunately, Lister's limited procedures were not sufficiently thorough. In the words of Nicholas M. Greene, they were "not adequate to allow surgeons to open infected joints or body cavities with impunity."[6] Even with the advance of "Listerism," hands were not scrubbed, surgeons wore street clothes, instruments were placed on unsterile towels, sponges were reused after being dipped in carbolic acid solution, etc.—with the result that surgeons using antiseptic methods could not demonstrate results significantly more favorable than surgeons not doing so. The American surgeon Samuel D. Gross observed in 1876 that "little, if any faith, is placed by any enlightened or experienced surgeon on this side of the Atlantic in the so-called carbolic acid treatment of Professor Lister, apart from the care which is taken in applying the dressing, or what is the same thing, in clearing away clots and excluding air from the wounds."[7] In the early 1880s, speakers at the American Surgical Association spoke, with rare exception, against Listerism, testifying that "neither they nor most other surgeons in their communities used antiseptic surgery."[8]

An appreciation for the "antiseptic conscience" gradually obtained. An increased understanding of infection— the chief problem was not germs in the air but germs on the body of the patient, the hands of the surgeon, and the surgical instruments—resulted in the use of steam and dry heat sterilization, the wearing of sterile gowns and masks, and the use of metal instruments. Antisepsis (using disinfectants during surgery to kill microorganisms) was replaced by asepsis (using sterile procedure to exclude microorganisms from the field of operation). With the additional discovery of the Xray in 1895, and the development of the sciences of physiology and pathology, "surgery was transformed from an act of desperation to a scientific method of dealing with illness."[9]

The number and kinds of surgeries subsequently increased. At the Massachusetts General Hospital, the number of operations annually averaged thirty-seven between 1841 and 1845 (the years immediately prior to Morton's successful demonstration of anesthesia), rose to ninety-eight between 1847 and 1851 (the years immediately following it), and reached thirty-seven hundred in 1898. By the end of the century surgery ceased to be superficial, expanding, for example, from amputations and excisions to intraabdominal interventions. Statistics gathered from Scotland, England, and Spain show a similar pattern in the rate of surgery increase as well as in the degree of complexity.[10]

Women

In 1873, three nurses' training schools were established in New York, New Haven, and Boston. The first such schools in the United

States, they signaled a change from lay nursing viewed as a menial, lower-class occupation (sometimes performed by women drafted from penitentiaries and almshouses) to that of a respectable profession. (There is, of course, a centuries-old commitment to nursing in various religious communities, both male and female.)[11] In his important study, *The Social Transformation of American Medicine*, Paul Starr points out that the movement toward nursing reform "originated, not with doctors, but among upper-class women, who had taken on the role of guardians of a new hygienic order. . . . Professional nursing . . . emerged neither from medical discoveries nor from a program of hospital reform initiated by physicians; outsiders saw the need first."[12]

The American schools were "Nightingale" schools, modeled after the St. Thomas Hospital Training School for Nurses founded in 1860 by Florence Nightingale. Gifts of money from a grateful public after her service in the Crimea were the source of funds for her school. Though the germ theory of disease was not yet understood when Nightingale labored at the British army hospital in Scutari (1854–1856), her emphasis on cleanliness, hygiene, and ventilation had proven dramatically successful: the death rate in the British military hospitals was reduced from 40 to 2 percent. She then turned her attention to the civilian hospital, declaring in her *Notes on Hospitals* (1857) that "as the very first requirement . . . it should do the sick no harm." Nightingale argued for a hospital environment that would be safe, that would "allow nature to work in the direction of health for the patient."[13] She went on to detail such things as "the number of patients under one roof, the space required between beds, bad sites and bad climates for hospital construction, and the potentials for defects in such things as ventilation, warming, drainage, kitchens, floors, laundries, furniture, bedding, the water supply, fuel, and the disposal of foul linen." Nightingale urged that hospital architecture be conducive to nursing efficiency, with "economy of attendance, ease of supervision, convenience as to the number of sick in the same ward and on the same floor . . . and sufficient accommodations for nurses to overlook their wards."[14] She also worked to standarize the naming and classification of diseases within hospitals, where formerly (pre-1859) each hospital had had its own method.

Starr notes that while some doctors approved of the American women philanthropists' desire to establish nurses' training schools that would attract "the wholesome daughters of the middle class," other medical men were not. Their concern was that "educated nurses would not do as they were told—a remarkable comment on the status anxieties of nineteenth-century physicians." But, like Florence Nightingale, "the women reformers did not depend on the physicians' approval." And "eventually, of course, physicians came not only to accept but to rely on trained nurses, who proved essential in carrying out the more complex work that hospitals were taking on."[15]

Of the contribution of professional nursing to the changing image of hospitals, the preeminent medical historian Richard Shyrock says:

All of this related to the public opinion of medical service in general, since the nurses came into more continuous contact with the patient than did any other figure in the whole range of medical personnel. Good nursing was invaluable from a technical point of view. It might make all the difference in the outcome of the individual case, and patients sometimes realized this. Better nursing was an essential feature in the gradual improvement of hospitals, and this in turn modified the earlier popular attitude toward these institutions. . . . The whole spirit of hospitals changed.[16]

An even stronger statement is made by Ellen Davidson Baer. In responding to a view that "defines medicine as so dominating a context that all others are dwarfed in its shadow," she poses the argument that "nursing made medicine look good":

Medicine's ultimate success, technological advances and subsequent impressive social power were achieved through hospitals, and nurses made those hospitals work. Nurses made them reasonable choices for sick-care, providing the environment in which patients felt safe enough to permit medical instrumentation to occur. The development of medical practice, education, therapeutics, et al proceeded from that point. Happily, one prominent physician understood that and reminded his contemporaries in 1910: "Now one must have some understanding of the value of the profession of nursing in modern medicine. . . . It has changed the face of modern medicine; it is revolutionary in its influence upon the progress of modern medicine."[17]

Anesthesia

"Most of the fatal cases can be traced to a careless administration of the remedy." (1859)
"At present it would not pay any one to devote all his time to giving anesthetics." (1899)[18]

A witness to the 1846 successful anesthesia demonstration, Henry J. Bigelow, later reflected on the significance of the event, saying that while various means of reducing surgical pain had been known for centuries, what had been lacking was an anesthetic that (1) would affect all similarly, (2) would consistently lead to insensibility to pain for a predetermined length of time, and (3) was safe.[19] It would, in fact, take many years beyond 1846 to begin to meet these requirements.

With the acceptance of asepsis and the emergence of professional nursing and hospital care, elements were in place for a removal of the remaining obstacle in the path of the advancement of surgery. Continuous and safe anesthesia delivery: it was a problem that had existed from the beginning of surgical anesthesia, but was only perceived with growing clarity as the problem of infection faded.

Early methods of surgical anesthesia were crude and dangerous. A handkerchief soaked in chloroform and clasped over a patient's nose would induce sleep quickly—perhaps a permanent sleep. Ether was administered with a sponge held over the patient's nose and mouth. The danger here was that since little air could pass through the wet sponge, the patient inhaling nearly pure ether vapor might get "ether pneumonia" and die. In any case he was likely to fight violently against the suffocation.

In 1859, a discussion of the dangers attending chloroform anesthesia included observations on the part of one doctor that "the danger from its use he considers to arise chiefly from the rash administration." The example then cited is one that would be echoed over the following decades:

In some cases Dr. M. had seen chloroform administered, by young gentlemen, rather in a careless manner; as they become interested in the operation, they are apt to apply the sponge too closely to the patient's nostrils, and thus prevent, to a great degree, the admixture of air with the vapor of the anesthetic. . . . In fact, he believed that most of the fatal cases can be traced to a careless administration of the remedy.[20]

At the end of the century—forty years later—the problem of careless administration of anesthetics was still being discussed. A recurring theme was that anesthesia duty continued to be assigned to the least experienced member of the staff:

Not infrequently, as all operators are aware, the life of the patient, no less than the success of the operation, is jeopardized by the careless or ignorant manner in which this important part of the procedure is carried out by a *novicus* just out of the medical school. In almost all institutions it is the junior on the staff, who is going through the process of gaining knowledge and skill rather than applying that previously acquired to whom this important duty is given over. (1897)[21]

And again:

Unfortunately, in most hospitals one of the younger internes is, as a rule, selected to administer the anaesthetic. The operator accustomed to having a novice give chloroform or ether for him is kept on the *qui vive* while performing the operation and watching the administration of the anaesthetic. Such a condition of affairs is not conducive to the best work of the surgeon. (1898)[22]

Since there were "many surgeons who are unwilling to share either the credit or the emoluments of their work," the anesthetizer suffered economically—another common theme. An additional irony was that the more dutiful and skillful the student-practitioner, the greater his risk of suffering professional disadvantage as well:

Then, too, it was not thought necessary to pay the anesthetizer anything; the surgeon took whatever fee was paid, considering that the privilege of assisting him and seeing how he did his work was ample reward for all the necessary assistants. In order to share in this benefit, the anesthetizer usually devoted more attention to the operation than he did to the patient. The student who cared to learn to operate—and what one did not?—avoided this assignment whenever possible. As accidents multiplied there came to be a feeling among some operators that perhaps a skilled man in this place might be an advantage. Then it became a positive disadvantage to a young man to get a reputation for skillful administration of anesthetics, for he was called upon oftener, his opportunities for learning surgery were lessened, *and still no one thought of offering him adequate pay for the time and skill required.* (1899) (emphasis added)[23]

Where anesthetizers *were* compensated, the practices were commonly "radically wrong and cannot result in anything but dissatisfaction to all parties concerned." For example, the anesthetizer might receive a small sum from an "operator," with the patient unaware of "how much, if anything," the anesthetizer received. The impression thus conveyed to the public is that the anesthetizer "and his work are of little if any importance":

For the operator to charge $100 or $200 for performing a simple uncomplicated operation and give the anesthetizer $5 for con-

ducting a difficult and complicated anesthesia, in which he has had
to exert all his energy and skill to keep the patient alive, is an
injustice which is not calculated to increase the number or efficiency
of anesthetizers.[24]

The even bolder practice of "ghost anesthesia" occurred:

> A patient stipulated to pay a surgeon $200 for performing an
> operation. He afterward requested that the most experienced anes-
> thetizer available be obtained to administer the anesthetic. The
> surgeon informed the patient that that would cost $25 additional,
> and the patient said he would gladly pay it. The surgeon employed
> a student to give the anesthetic, collected $225, gave the student $5
> and thus received $220 for the operation.[25]

With the lack of financial and professional incentives for physicians
to specialize in anesthetics, some looked to draw practitioners from
more marginal medical ranks. Thus one surgeon reflected in 1897
that, "I have often wondered why some of the young medical men,
who act as agents for proprietary medicine firms, wholesale drug
houses and publishers do not select a by far more honorable calling,
and make this a specialty."[26]

Years earlier, other surgeons had quietly turned to the religious
hospital Sister. For work that required complete attention to the well-
being of the patient, contentment with patient care as an end in itself,
and acceptance of the gravest responsibility without economic reward,
it was a wise choice.

Early Nurse Anesthetists

In 1941, Agatha C. Hodgins, the founder of the American Association of Nurse Anesthetists voiced a wish: "While we would all like to
know with certainty the name of the first nurse anesthetist, so that we
might give to her prior honor, we reluctantly admit there still remains
a veil of mystery over this lady."[27] A few years later, Virginia S.
Thatcher researched a history of nurse anesthetists, discovering the
significant contribution of the religious nursing Sisters to professional
anesthesia care. Thatcher was able to draw aside that "veil of mystery"
because these women, who lived and worked in self-effacing
obscurity, paradoxically led lives more well-documented than most—
certainly more than most other nineteenth-century women. Canon
law requirements resulted in detailed records of individual nuns.
"The majority of repositories . . . normally include their applications

for admission or records of their entrance, formation, and profession. They may also contain birth dates and places, places of baptism and confirmation, and information on education and family background; nearly all have complete necrologies, and most take note of departures and dismissals from the ranks. Other typical records include lists of sisters' assignments and their elections; correspondence with the hierarchy and with sister communities; chronicles of various foundations and ministries; and financial statements and account books. Many also contain members' diaries, unpublished memoirs."[28]

Thatcher's inquiries to religious houses yielded not only the identity of Sister Mary Bernard, who was called upon to take up anesthetist's duties within a year of entering St. Vincent's Hospital, Erie, Pennsylvania, in 1877, and thereby emerged as the first identifiable nurse anesthetist, but of some fifty other Sisters who took up the work in the last two decades of the century. Acknowledging her evidence to be inevitably "fragmentary," Thatcher viewed these figures as giving "only . . . a glimpse of what was undoubtedly a prevailing practice in many Catholic hospitals."[29]

A tantalizing "glimpse" of secular practice is provided in the *1893* textbook of pioneering nursing educator, Isabel Adams Hampton Robb: *Nursing: Its Principles and Practices for Hospital and Private Use.* In it, she devotes an entire chapter to "The Administration of Anaesthetics," noting that "A nurse is often called upon in private practice to administer an anaesthetic."[30]

The scope of the *documented* contribution of the religious nursing-Sisters can be illustrated by focusing on only one of the communities. Two Sisters of the Third Order of the Hospital Sisters of St. Francis from Muenster, Germany, established a community in Springfield, Illinois, in November, 1875; on June 22, 1879, they dedicated their St. John's Hospital. "There, in 1880, the administration of chloroform and ether was taught by the surgeons to Sister Aldonza Eltrich (1860–1920), a frail nun who did lace work when not occupied with anesthesia. Also, that year Sister Vanossa Woenke was trained as an anesthetist." Between 1884 and 1888, the Missouri Pacific Railroad established five hospitals for its employees in Illinois and Missouri, which the Hospital Sisters of the Third Order of St. Francis managed, and in which their Sisters continued to serve as anesthetists.[31] In 1912 Mother Magdalene Wiedlocher, herself an anesthetist, organized a course in anesthesia at St. John's Hospital for Sisters who were graduate nurses; in 1924 the postgraduate courses were opened to secular nurses. One of the results of Thatcher's recovery of this history was the conferring by the American Association of Nurse Anesthetists of its "Award of Appreciation" to the Hospital Sisters of the Third Order of St. Francis, Springfield, Illinois, in 1954.

Of course, other communities of both Catholic and Protestant nursing-Sisters figured in the late–nineteenth century professionalization of anesthesia delivery. Thatcher's catalogue not only recognizes their service, but provides another "glimpse" of anesthesia practice:

At the Mercy Hospital in Chicago, Sister Mary Ethelreda O'Dwyer from Bausha, Tipperary, learned from the illustrious surgeon John Benjamin Murphy (1857–1916) how to drop ether in 1891, and the skill of this Sister of Mercy with the open-drop technic brought fame to the Mercy Hospital. In 1891 Sister Peter Chrysologus Crevier of the Sisters of Charity of Montreal began to give anesthetics at the Providence Hospital in Seattle. Other Sisters of the Order also took up the work during the last decade of the nineteenth century: in 1896 Sister Andrew Moreau (d. 1945) at St. Vincent's Hospital, Portland, Ore.; in 1896 Sister Emery Lalonde (d. 1943) at St. Patrick's Hospital, Missoula, Mont.; in 1897 Sister Mary Vincent Brown (d. 1933) at St. Mary's Hospital, Astoria, Ore.; in 1898 Sister Oswald Dorion (d. 1919) at St. Patrick's Hospital, Missoula, Mont.; and in 1899 Sister Mary Gregory Jutras (d. 1945) at Sacred Heart Hospital, Spokane, Wash.

From the Order of the Sisters of Mercy, Baltimore, the first to be assigned to anesthesia was Sister Mary Celestine Doyle (d. 1944), who, in 1893, began her work at the Mercy Hospital in Baltimore. In 1896 at St. Joseph's Hospital in Denver, Sister Mary Gonzaga O'Connell (d. 1939) of the Sisters of Charity of Leavenworth took up her duties as anesthetist. That same year Sister Mary Ignatius Kerns (d. 1919) of the Sisters of Mercy of Chicago began to give anesthetics at the Mercy Hospital in Davenport, Iowa. In 1897 Sister Martha Lawler (1871–1935) of the Daughters of Charity of St. Vincent de Paul was trained in anesthesia at the Troy Hospital, Troy, N.Y., by the chief surgeon, Dr. Harvey, and embarked upon a career as anesthetist and teacher of anesthetists that took her to St. Joseph's Hospital, Chicago, Mary's Help Hospital, San Francisco, and Charity Hospital, New Orleans. Sister Mary Antonia Cawley of the Sisters of Mercy of Wilkes-Barre served as the first anesthetist of that Order at the Mercy Hospital, Wilkes-Barre, when it opened in 1898. From the Sisters of St. Joseph, Nazareth, Mich., Sister Mary Constance began to give anesthetics at Borgess Hospital, Kalamazoo, Mich., in 1898, after a special course in anesthesia at St. Elizabeth's Hospital, Chicago. Perhaps even earlier, two of the Franciscan Sisters of the Sacred Heart, Joliet, Ill.—Sister Mary Ida (d. 1939), who entered the Order in 1872, and Sister Mary Georgia (d. 1919), who entered in 1873—were administering anesthesia at St.

Francis Hospital, Freeport, Ill., and at St. Joseph's Hospital, Joliet, the dates of their assignments antedating the records of the Order.

Among the Protestant as well as Catholic nursing orders nurse anesthetists were to be found during the 1890s. In 1897 at the Lutheran Deaconess Hospital in Minneapolis, Sister Lena Nelson gained experience in administering anesthesia before going to Austin, Minn., to carry on the work, and Sister Marie S. Anderson, who entered the Lutheran Diaconate at Omaha in 1895, began to give anesthetics in 1898 at Dr. Dearborn's Hospital in Wakefield, Neb.[32]

Perhaps the most touching figure in Thatcher's narrative of this period is that of Sister Secundina Mindrup (1868–1951), one of the Hospital Sisters of the Third Order of St. Francis. Called "Secundina" because she entered the convent twice (the first time at the age of twelve, played with dolls, and had to be sent home), she lived to communicate her memories to Thatcher: "The doctors would come with their assistants to give the anesthesia, but then they would need the assistant for something else and would teach the Sister how to give the anesthesia." In the 1880s, "Sister Secundina devised her own method for judging when more ether or chloroform or alcohol-chloroform-ether mixture should be given—a decade of prayers on her rosary and it was time to give a little more. In an apron with two split pockets she carried everything that anyone in the hospital might want, and in one of the pockets she secreted a bottle of chloroform. This she quietly and judiciously used to supplement the ether anesthesia when the surgeon required more relaxation."[33] Another memorable figure is that of Sister Lawrence Niehoff, of the same order, who began her anesthesia in 1890: "Sister Lawrence first assisted at operations by helping to hold the instruments; she was taught to give anesthetics when a physician who came from Litchfield, Ill., to perform this service expressed a desire to learn more about surgery. When the occasion demanded, Sister Lawrence would put two patients to sleep at once. Placed with their heads together, first one and then the other would be anesthetized, and then she would sit on a stool between the two heads and watch them both."[34]

A memoir from one of these women, Sister Marie S. Anderson of the Lutheran Diaconate at Omaha, was published in 1941. She recalled her initiation into the field in 1898:

After my training was completed in Omaha, it was decided that I should take charge of a small private hospital in a little country town. As the doctor who owned the hospital did his own surgery, and as I was the only nurse, it fell to my lot to take care of the patients, prepare the operating room and give the anesthetic, so I had to learn something about it quickly. Dr. B. B. Davis hurriedly gave me brief instructions. He told me the signs of anesthesia and how to administer the ether, then performed the emergency abdominal operation and I carried the patient through safely, but I was happy when the patient was awake again. I nursed her until she left the hospital, and we became good friends. . . —a joy to me because it was my first experience in anesthesia.

Moved by compassion for her patients, Sister Marie sought ways to ease their discomfort and to allay their fears. As did other early anesthetists, she experimented on herself, making a parallel discovery to improve technique:

While engaged in bedside nursing, I often heard patients say: "I am not afraid of the operation, but I do dread the anesthetic." My sympathy grew ever stronger and I longed to take away that fear if I could. So I began experimenting by placing the ether mask over my face, just as we did when administering the ether to the patient. My reaction showed me how the patient must feel—it was a suffocating, breath-taking experience. As a result I began the practice of holding the mask away from the face at first, gradually letting it down as the patient became accustomed to breathing ether vapor. My new technique won the patients and was favored by other anesthetists and it was soon in common use, descriptions of the method appearing in the literature on anesthesia at that period.

After a forty-four-year career in anesthesia, she could claim a record of thousands of anesthetics "without a single death on the operating table."[35]

Alice Magaw: "The Mother of Anesthesia"

Apart from their own anesthesia work, the Sisters of St. Francis were to play a further role in the development of anesthesia care. It was their Rochester, Minnesota, community that established St. Mary's Hospital in 1889 on the condition that Dr. William Worrell Mayo take charge of it. It would soon become a gathering place for those interested in learning techniques from its brilliant surgeons. Visitors would also see "peerless"[36] administration of anesthetics at the hands of Alice Magaw and other nurse anesthetists of Mayo Clinic.

As sketched above, early methods of surgical anesthesia were crude and dangerous. Barbarity was still a common feature of the operating room:

The patient was anaesthetized by being placed on the table, a broad leather strap passed over the abdomen and another one over the legs, both tightly belted to the table. The narcotizer having prepared a cone made of a newspaper, stuffed it with either cotton or cheesecloth on which we had poured the entire contents of a 100-gram can of ether. Placing a towel over the patient's eyes, he slipped the cone over the patient's mouth and nose, then motioned to the orderly and nurse who were standing by to throw their weight on the arms and legs of the victim and the battle was on. The patient struggled, the concentration of the anaesthetic induced spasm, and in the middle of the flight the poor victim crowed like a rooster with an attack of the whooping cough.[37]

New devices were being designed for better administration of anesthesia; in the early years, this meant *dropping* rather than *pouring* chloroform and ether. James Young Simpson, around 1860, dropped chloroform onto a single layer of cloth laid over the patient's nose and mouth. Use of a chloroform bottle with a drop tube attachment controlling its flow onto a small fabric-covered wire frame held over the patient's face was described by Thomas Skinner in 1862. Skinner's mask was especially popular in Germany, which had assumed a leadership role in surgery by quickly embracing the principle of asepsis as well as the need for research in chemistry and physics. It was a German surgeon, Johannes Friedrich August von Esmarch, who designed a simplified Skinner mask around 1879.

The open-drop method and Esmarch mask made their way to the Mayo Clinic—though the route is unclear. Like so many areas of the history of anesthesia, priority is debated. James E. Moore, the Minneapolis surgeon, recalled that Alice Magaw

gives me credit for having brought to this country the drop method. I never made any claim to that credit. In 1885 I went to Germany, and while there I had an extensive experience that I could not have here. . . . [From Berlin] I brought ["an anesthetizer skilled in the use of chloroform by the drop method"] with me in 1886, and he remained here nearly a year. He gave my anesthetics, and I was pleased to loan him all about. I wrote this up for publication, and Dr. Mayo says he learned the use of the drop method from that.[38]

Elsewhere, Magaw recollected:

During the past six years I have acted as anaesthetist in the service of the Drs. Mayo, at St. Mary's Hospital. In a general way the anaesthesia has been conducted under the direction of Dr. A. W.

Stinchfield, or in his absence, by Dr. Christopher Graham. . . . [We] finally fell into the use of the Esmarch mask and drop method introduced in the Augustana Hospital [Chicago] by Dr. L. H. Prince in the service of Dr. [Albert J.] Ochsner.[39]

Whether it was Dr. Moore of Minneapolis or the close relationship of the Mayos with Dr. Ochsner that brought the technique to the Clinic (according to Dr. George W. Crile, "In those days Will [Mayo] and [Albert] Ochsner were inseparable friends"[40]), in the hands of their nurses it became an art.

What was initially a matter of necessity for the Mayos became a matter of choice: "In the first place . . . they had no interns. And when the interns came, the brothers decided that a nurse was better suited to the task because she was more likely to keep her mind strictly on it, whereas the intern was naturally more interested in what the surgeon was doing."[41] The Clinic's first nurse anesthetists were two Rochester sisters, Dinah and Edith Graham, both graduates of the School of Nursing at the Women's Hospital in Chicago. The five Sisters of St. Francis on the staff took over all nursing and housekeeping duties, while the Grahams, trained by William W. Mayo, administered the anesthesia and performed general office and secretarial work. Dinah's tenure was brief; Edith continued until her marriage to Charles H. Mayo in 1893. Her friend, Alice Magaw (1860–1928), another Rochester girl who graduated from the Women's Hospital, Chicago, succeeded her. So brilliant was her work that, as Mayo biographer Helen Clapesattle has noted, she "won more widespread notice than that of any other member of the Rochester group apart from the brothers."[42]

As a nurse, Magaw could not be a member of a medical society. Her first talks were occasioned by invitations from the Olmsted County Medical Society; they were then published in state medical journals. Also, because she was a nurse, her papers are not listed in the *Physicians of the Mayo Clinic* bibliography. One Magaw study, however, was included in the *Collected Papers by the Staff of St. Mary's Hospital, Mayo Clinic, Rochester, Minnesota, 1905–1909*. When this 1906 paper was reprinted in the *Bulletin of the National Association of Nurse Anesthetists*, in 1939, it is not surprising that it was incorrectly identified as "the first paper published by a nurse anesthetist."[43] There was no awareness of her earlier work. This is of considerable significance for the history of nursing. As historian Gerda Lerner has pointed out, "The cataloguing and indexing of manuscripts have great impact on defining themes and sources of importance in historical scholarship. The major papers of historical figures, which have been preserved, catalogued, and indexed and thus made available through long-range projects financed by public grants, are skewed by patriarchal bias and consign women to the limbo of historical nonexistence."[44] Fortunately, Clapesattle catalogued Magaw's papers in 1941.[45]

"Observations in Anesthesia," a report on over three thousand cases, was published in the *Northwestern Lancet* in 1899. It was Magaw's first publication. In 1900, she updated the year's work in "Observations on 1092 cases of anesthesia from Jan. 1, 1899 to Jan. 1, 1900" in the *St. Paul Medical Journal:* "She used the Esmarch mask with two thicknesses of stockinette; she had both ether and chloroform ready to give, whichever was indicated by the condition of the patient. Six hundred and seventy-four operations were performed with ether, 245 with chloroform and 173 with a mixture of the two, *without an accident, the need for artificial respiration or the occurrence of pneumonia or any serious results.* By 1904 the total had grown to 11,000 and by 1906 to over 14,000 without a death directly attributable to the anesthesia."[46]

In her 1906 paper, "A Review of Over Fourteen Thousand Surgical Anesthesias," Magaw emphasized that other anesthetic techniques had been tried, but were found to be less satisfactory than the "open method" of ether:

> We have tried almost all methods advocated that seemed at all reasonable, such as nitrous oxide gas as a preliminary to ether (this method was used in one thousand cases), a mixture of scopolamine and morphine as a preliminary to ether in 73 cases, also chloroform and ether, and have found them to be very unsatisfactory, if not harmful, and have returned to ether "drop method" each time, which method we have used for over ten years.[47]

Magaw stressed the need for the anesthetist to be sensitive to the unique needs of each patient. For example:

> It is a mistake to think that the same elevation of the head will do for all patients. . . . All jaws cannot be handled in the same manner. . . . The dose required for each individual patient cannot be estimated so as to be of any value, as it depends largely on the temperament of the patient, pathologic condition present, time consumed in anesthetizing and operating.[48]

For Magaw, it was the *experience* of the anesthetist in reading and reacting quickly to the condition of the patient that was of the greatest importance: "It is far better for the anesthetist to become skillful in watching for symptoms and preventing them, than to become so proficient in the use of" such articles as "an oxygen-tank, a loaded hypodermic syringe, or tongue-forceps."[49] At the same time she acknowledged that experienced anesthetists were scarce: "There is no class of work that has so little encouragement, and few are willing to follow this line of work (that, in difficulty and nerve strain, is next to that of a surgeon) long enough to become familiar with the first requirements of a good anesthetizer."[50]

A significant element of Magaw's success resulted from her attention to the psychological dimension of the anesthetic experience. The Mayos had begun with the practice, common to other hospitals, of anesthetizing patients in an area adjoining the operating room. The theory was that patients would be less agitated if they did not see all the accompaniments of surgery, and were brought into the operating room only when unconscious. It became apparent to the Mayos, however, that moving a relaxed patient from one room to another, with possibly variant temperatures, could contribute to respiratory complications. They therefore began the practice of anesthetizing patients in the operating room.

A surprise benefit was that the operating room activity provided a *positive* distraction for the patient. As Magaw explained:

> During the thirteen years' work at St. Mary's Hospital all patients have been anesthetized on the operating table in the operating room, and preparation of the patient was going on at the same time. Experience has taught us that preparation of the patient while going under the anesthetic is one of the important factors in producing a rapid surgical narcosis; for it diverts his attention, *and much less anesthetic is required.* It matters not in what position the patient must be for operation, we fix him accordingly, and the preparation is begun at the same time as the anesthetic, and we feel certain that this procedure enables us to hasten narcosis.[51] (emphasis added)

Magaw's discussion of "suggestion," "the subconscious or secondary self," and "suggestive influence" avoided the term "hypnotic suggestion," though other writers would use it in connection with the Mayo technique, and on at least one occasion Dr. Charles Mayo elaborated on this component. Magaw wrote:

> Suggestion is a great aid in producing a comfortable narcosis. The anesthetist must be able to inspire confidence in the patient, and a great deal depends on the manner of approach. One must be quick to notice the temperament, and decide which mode of suggestion will be the most effective in the particular case: the abrupt, crude, and very firm, or the reasonable, sensible, and natural. The latter

mode is far the best in the majority of cases. The subconscious or secondary self is particularly susceptible to suggestive influence; therefore, during the administration, the anesthetist should make those suggestions that will be most pleasing to this particular subject. Patients should be prepared for each stage of the anesthesia with an explanation of just how the anesthetic is expected to affect him; "talk him to sleep," *with the addition of as little ether as possible.*[52] (emphasis added)

Two years earlier, in a discussion with his colleagues after Magaw presented another of her papers, Dr. Charles Mayo commented:

There is one point I wish to speak of, and that is the question of hypnotism as an anesthetic. Very frequently one goes into a large hospital, and finds that the anesthetic is given in an adjoining room by an interne. These patients come to a certain surgeon, as a rule, because they have confidence in him, after he has examined them personally, previous to the operation, and decided what is best to do, they keep confidence in him or they do not stay for the operation. When he sends them away with an interne into an adjoining room to have the anesthetic given it excites their fear, but if he is in the room it gives them confidence because of his presence. The next thing is suggestion. We have done a little of it, but always with anesthesia. When the drunk of anesthesia comes on, or when it passes off, the patient is extremely ready to receive suggestion, and the anesthetizer who attempts to give an anesthetic to a patient and says, "Keep still; don't do that now; keep on breathing," and so on, will find his patient struggling and talking right along. It is just like antagonizing a drunken man. It arouses a spirit of antagonism and he keeps up his struggles. You give an anesthetic in from five to ten minutes and say, "You are all right; your pulse is good; keep right on breathing," and you do not have to say it loud. It is for the ear of the patient alone, and you will have no difficulty in controlling your patient.[53]

An interesting, early application of these insights was an important part of the work of the Minneapolis surgeon, Robert Emmett Farr, one of the few twentieth-century American surgeons who used local or regional anesthesia with small children. Dr. Roderick K. Calverley has noted the critical role of the anesthetist in the success of this approach: "Farr stressed his dependence on the support of an anesthetist by giving her an unique title. Even when supplemental inhalation anesthesia was not required, his 'psycho-anesthetist' comforted and diverted his younger patients," contributing to the favorable outcome of the surgery.[54]

Medical people came from around the country—and the world—to observe the technique of Mayo's nurse anesthetists. An Iowa doctor said of their expertise and influence: "Many of us have had the pleasure and privilege of seeing that peerless anesthetist, Alice Magaw, and also Miss [Florence] Henderson, who anesthetizes for Dr. Charles Mayo, 'talk their patients to sleep,' and we have been charmed and instructed by the manner in which these ladies do their work. The lessons they have taught, and are teaching, practitioners have been carried far and wide, and practiced by men throughout Iowa and many other states."[55]

Not only were the techniques of the nurse anesthetists disseminated, but the practice of training nurses for the work also spread. Dr. J. M. Baldy, a vocal supporter of nurse anesthetists, described the shift in thinking at The Gynecean Hospital, Philadelphia:

The time-honored custom in hospitals of utilizing the junior resident physician in this capacity [of anesthetist] has proven itself not only a failure, but a disaster in many instances. The equally unscientific use of the nearest practising physician in surgery in private houses has proved itself similarly unfit. . . . The perfect solution, of course, would be a medical man of a high grade of intelligence, with a well-grounded medical and surgical education, a special education in anesthetics supplemented by a natural inclination in this direction as against any other. Are the attractions of anesthesia sufficient to overcome the disadvantages of the scientific narrowness and lack of opportunity for distinction and income to hold a sufficient number of men of this type or even of great worth in this field? The answer seems apparent. . . . The Gynecean Hospital of Philadelphia has now had a graduate nurse in charge of its anesthesia (independent of all aid) for a year. . . . My proposal originally was met by the universal opposition of everyone connected with the hospital. . . . A nurse about to graduate was selected and turned over to the anesthetist (a physician . . .) for instruction during the remaining months of her nursing course. . . . The result has been to win without exception the approval of everyone about the institution. . . . We note in a recent report of St. Mary's Hospital, Rochester, Minn., that the Mayo Clinic has four official anesthetists—all women. It was in this clinic we were first impressed with the capacity of a woman in this position.[56]

This scenario was much-repeated as nurse anesthesia spread from a heavy concentration in the Midwest to the Eastern states.[57]

"Notes on the Administration of Anesthetics in America, with Special Reference to the Practice at the Mayo Clinic," a paper presented by Mrs. Dickinson-Berry, M.D., to the Section of Anaesthetics of the Royal Society of Medicine in 1912, reflects the international reputation of the Mayo nurse anesthetists.[58] It is of special interest because it is a commonplace in histories of anesthesia written from the physician point of view that, unlike the situation in Britain, anesthesia in this country suffered because physicians were slow to embrace it as a specialty. Nurse anesthetists are seen as having impeded progress, rather than having contributed to it.

Dickinson-Berry's paper, and the discussion following its presentation, indicate that some British physician-anesthetists felt they had things to learn from the Mayo nurse anesthetists. There is an additional irony here in that Dickinson-Berry begins her presentation with what she calls a "cursory glimpse" of other anesthetists she observed in the United States. The first mentioned is the brilliant pioneering physician-anesthetist, James T. Gwathmey, noted here also as "President of a recently formed Society of Anaesthetists"; Dickson-Berry devotes eight sentences to his methods. She then continues:

I now come to what was one of the main objects of my tour in America, the visit to Rochester, Minnesota. Like most people, I had heard and read much of the excellence of the anaesthetics at the Mayo clinic. In the last paper I read on the subject before leaving England the writer was inclined to attribute this partly to an inborn faculty for administering anaesthetics on the part of women, and partly to the aid of hypnotic suggestion. I was therefore very glad to have the opportunity of seeing them myself.[59]

Again, we are told that "the patient is talked to soothingly all the time":

There was seldom any trouble during the first stage of anaesthesia, the anaesthetist continued to talk to the patient, describing in an encouraging manner the process of going under and assuring him he was taking the anaesthetic well. During the second stage there was frequently a little coughing and occasionally some excitement, but rarely any troublesome struggling. . . . Though the anaesthesia was often very light the anaesthetists always had the patients well in hand, and I never saw actual struggling or vomiting, though occasionally slight attempts at retching might occur.[60]

Dickinson-Berry and her colleagues agree that the "open ether method in America" was different from that practiced in Britain:

The essential feature of the open ether method in America was the absolutely continuous administration; a drop on the mask every two seconds was the rate. In fact, at Rochester it was called the "drop method." In this country the anaesthetist would often pour 2 dr. or 3 dr. on the mask, then stop for a few minutes and then pour a few more drachms on the mask. This was not open ether as practised in America.[61]

"Ether by the open method with the skill exhibited at Rochester," said Dickinson-Berry, "requires much practice."[62]

In what is, in effect, another chapter in the chauvinistic "Great Trans-Atlantic Debate" over the relative merits of ether versus chloroform anesthesia—with the former the general favorite in the United States, and the latter preferred in Britain—*the safety of the lightness of the ether anesthesia of the Mayo nurse anesthetists* becomes the center of this British-physician discussion. In her various papers, Magaw had noted that chloroform, though an easier anesthetic from the viewpoint of the surgeon and anesthetist (herself included), was *not* safer for the patient:

For the sake of the patient my preference is for ether; for myself, I would say, like most anaesthetizers, that I would prefer giving chloroform, as we escape so many of the unpleasant things that naturally follow the use of ether.[63]

After Dickinson-Berry's report on her visit to Mayo Clinic, the President of the Section of Anaesthetics reflected:

The most striking difference [between British and American anesthetic practice] appeared to him to be the slighter degree of narcosis which was considered necessary in America. The description of the return in stomach cases almost to consciousness, which the surgeon not only permitted but desired, showed what a difference there was in the practice of the two countries. *Evidently in the States safety was the first consideration.*[64] (emphasis added)

Another respondent observed:

The most important conclusion from the paper . . . was that in States light anaesthesia was adopted *because of its safety.* The belief in England that deep anaesthesia prevented shock was dying out, but it had been the greatest handicap, and had caused more accidents in this country than anything else.[65] (emphasis added)

For discussant H. J. Paterson, "the reason the Americans had been so successful was that they had learned from us, while we, on our part, had not learned anything like so much from them."

> Nothing impressed him so much during his visit to America as the advantages of the open ether method as given at the Mayo clinic. Many years ago, in the exuberance of his surgical youth, he was rash enough to say, at the Medico-Chirurgical Society, that it was criminal for a surgeon to do an abdominal section under ether. Somebody in Rochester had read that remark, and when he went there he was asked to open a discussion on anaesthetics from the surgical point of view, in the expectation that he would be an advocate of chloroform. But he had been so impressed with the results of open ether that he thought he ought first to find out something of what went on behind the scenes. Therefore he spent a week in going round to all the patients who had had anaesthetics during the previous fortnight, examined their charts, made notes on them, asked questions about their sensations, and so on. When he came to open the discussion, he had to confess that he had been convinced of the superiority of open ether over chloroform for general surgery. Since he had returned home he had had all the more reason to remain assured that the opinion he had formed in Rochester as to the value of ether was correct.[66]

Finally, there is the lament that the British surgeons are less supportive of their anesthetists than surgeons in the United States. The resultant frustration concerning matters of patient safety is poignantly expressed (a British epithet for the anesthetist was "the Coroner's familiar"), and underscores the lack of meaningful status for the British *physician* anesthetists vis à vis British surgeons: "It seemed evident from the [Dickinson-Berry] paper that the anaesthetists in America in their use of ether had the whole of the profession at their back. Nothing could be done in the education of the general public on this matter unless the support of the profession was behind the opinion of the anaesthetists. So long as patients could answer one's recommendations by saying there were so many other kinds of anaesthetic in use, and would prefer one of the others, it would be impossible to press the use of this, the best and safest form of anaesthesia. If it could be stated by surgeons that ether given by modern methods was thirty times safer than other forms of anaesthesia, though it might cause more inconvenience during the operation, the result would be that many more proposed operations would receive the patient's consent."[67]

What the above paper and discussion suggest—a less than ideal situation for British anesthetists and their patients—becomes inverted in physician-oriented histories of American practice. It seems as though a desired conclusion—that because anesthesia in Britain was a physician practice, it was intrinsically superior to anesthesia in the United States, where nurse anesthetists were permitted to practice, and physician-specialists came late to the field—is attached to contrary evidence. Thus, for example, in *Anesthesiology and The University*, Dr. Nicholas M. Greene notes the negative characteristics of chloroform (while noninflammable, it is less safe than ether, it depresses respiration, has histotoxic properties, and "increases the irritability of the heart and sensitizes it to arrhythmias, including fatal ventricular fibrillation"), as well as reasons why it nevertheless remained the British anesthetic of choice ("esthetic" properties, which Magaw had also acknowledged, as well as chauvinism, "a reluctance to accept as better anything, ether included, which came from a country as young and brash as the United States, so recently a colony"). From this Greene draws the remarkable conclusion:

> It became apparent to most physicians in Britain that chloroform was acceptable but far from ideal. Chloroform was associated with real dangers, and anesthesia was not to be entered into lightly or inadvisedly, an attitude many decades off in the United States. In the United Kingdom, chloroform anesthesia was, from the outset, administered only by physicians. For one hundred years British anesthetists held technical and clinical superiority over their American nurse counterparts.[68]

Martin Pernick has put a particularly cynical twist on Greene's argument, suggesting that "Critics charged that British physicians preferred chloroform over ether because the greater danger of the former agent ensured it would remain under professional (physician) control."[69]

In any case, Greene articulates an element of the physician-anesthetist Creation Myth that traces positive developments in anesthesia to a physician origin, and denies the nurse anesthetist contribution to the founding of the field. Others, however, did acknowledge that contribution, among them Dr. Charles H. Mayo, who titled nurse anesthetist Alice Magaw, "Mother of Anesthesia."

· 2 ·

Up Against That Sort of Thing

I n 1936, one of America's greatest surgeons said of nurse anesthetists: "I think this movement is one of the most beneficent movements we have seen in the whole field of operative surgery."[1] The speaker was George W. Crile, renowned for his research in the treatment of surgical shock. He recalled that earlier in his career he had faced a twofold problem with anesthetics. First, although developments in anesthesia and asepsis provided a new generation of surgeons a foundation for building a "remarkably efficient surgical practice," "there still remained a great task, viz., the reclamation of a large group of [health-handicapped] patients that constituted the tables of mortality if operated upon, and if unoperated they remained unrelieved or died."[2] Crile therefore sought a more subtle form of anesthesia.

He also sought a more subtle anesthetist than the intern: "I would like to state a fact that you probably do not know . . . that is how ill adapted an intern anesthetist was, and nearly all surgeons have arrived at this same conclusion. The intern was interested in his career—anesthesia was not his primary interest." Crile looked for an essential quality of "finesse," and found it, as the Mayos had, in the trained nurse: "I could see no other way out of the difficulty but to look about and consider all the nurses I knew and to choose from among those one who had the ideal qualities to undertake a great responsibility."[3] His choice was Agatha Cobourg Hodgins, a nurse with "a very interesting personality,"[4] who proved herself to be not only a brilliant anesthetist, but a woman of vision. She appreciated the significance of this development for professional nursing, and dedicated herself to establishing a national association committed to assuring a quality education for those nurses who entered the field.

Born in Toronto in 1877 to prosperous, conservative parents, she lead a sheltered early life. Rather than continue in a traditional path,

39

she chose after graduation from junior college to travel to the United States to enter the Boston City Hospital Training School for Nurses at the age of twenty-one. A report from the school described her as being "quiet and self-possessed in manner. She proves herself to be intelligent, amiable, and well bred. She is happy in her work and seems well adapted for the care of children. . . . Miss Hodgins might be considered an excellent nurse. She has always done her best. She is punctual, frank, tidy, and very patient."[5]

After graduation in 1900, she followed two of her classmates to Cleveland to work as head nurses in the private pavilion at Lakeside Hospital. Although her peers saw in her no mark of future greatness, George Crile said he "recognized in her the person who should be asked to take this responsibility" of anesthesia work:[6] "One morning in 1908 while making rounds I drew Miss Hodgins aside and presented to her what amounted to an annunciation. She had received no warning whatever about the plan to make her my special anesthetist, but she told me promptly that she would undertake it if I would remember always that she was giving her best."[7] Elsewhere he added: "I knew then I was not to find fault or scold. As a matter of fact, she need not have told me that because there never was a moment in all the episodes in our early experiences when I had any occasion to be disappointed in her work for even a moment."[8]

Their work began with animals: "We went up to the laboratory and gave anesthetics to animals; saw the good effects, the bad effects; the later effects."[9] Crile continued: "In order that [Miss Hodgins] might become familiar with the symptoms of death, I started her to work administering anesthetics to rabbits and dogs. From anesthetizing rabbits, she learned to anesthetize young babies. Her skill in amusing them with toys or my watch while she allowed the gas to play gently near the child's face until the sandman closed his eyes and he slipped back on the pillow was extraordinary."[10] This, for Crile, was the embodiment of "finesse."

Hodgins learned from additional sources. A colleague later recalled: "She read all that she could find on the subject and broadened her clinical knowledge in every way possible. Night after night she walked the wards where she listened to the sleeping patients' breathing in order that she might detect subtle differences."[11] She also joined the numbers of those who traveled to the Mayo Clinic to observe the technique of open-drop ether.

But the anesthetic technique that Lakeside Hospital would become celebrated for was nitrous oxide-oxygen. In his shock research, Crile had noted the "deleterious effects" of ether and chloroform anesthesia. It was through the work of two dentists—Dr. John Stephan and Dr. Charles K. Teter—that Crile found an alternative:

Dr. Teter had acquired a splendid empirical knowledge of the administration of nitrous oxide in his dental work and had invented an excellent apparatus bearing his name. A few administrations of this anesthetic by him for patients of mine were sufficient to indicate to me its clinical possibilities in my field, so I undertook a research in 1906 to ascertain if nitrous oxide gave better protection to the central nervous system than ether or chloroform.[12]

Crile's hypothesis was that nitrous oxide, with the addition of oxygen "to prevent the asphyxiating effects of too prolonged administration of this anesthetic agent," and "in the hands of a skilled anesthetist" could be used safely in major operations and thus become the anesthetic of choice.[13]

Crile now had his anesthetic and his anesthetist, with the result that, "From the very first day that I stole her from the pavilion, the work developed rapidly."[14] Interestingly, in this case it was the surgeon, not the anesthetist, who reported the results to various medical groups—perhaps underlining the unique situation that existed for Magaw at Mayo Clinic, which allowed a nurse to speak at physician gatherings. Crile recalled:

In 1909 I was able to report before the Southern Surgical and Gynecological Association that Miss Hodgins had administered nitrous oxide in 575 major operations, and in August 1911, I reported before the American Surgical Association, 10,787 surgical operations performed by me under either ether, or nitrous oxide supplemented by ether with no anesthetic death. I reported also the use of morphine and scopolamine as adjuncts to ether or nitrous oxide anesthesia in over three thousand operations.[15]

Yet Crile, the surgeon addressing his peers, did acknowledge the crucial role of his anesthetist/nurse:

The administering of an anesthetic is not only an art but a gift. In my mind it ranks close to the work of the operating surgeon. The nitrous oxide expert, for instance, must develop an anesthetic intuition. Oxygen is a pilot light to keep the flame of life burning safely. If the light burns too high, the patient immediately comes out from the anesthesia, if too low, the patient dies. Yet with a steady flow of gas under constant pressure, the patient is carried easily through the narrow zone of anesthesia. Miss Hodgins made an outstanding anesthetist for she had to a marked degree both the intelligence and the gift.[16]

Just as visitors came to Mayo Clinic and Alice Magaw to learn open-drop ether, so too they came to Lakeside for the nitrous oxide-oxygen technique:

That first year both Dr. George Brewer and Dr. Charles Frazier sent a nurse to Miss Hodgins to be trained. Visiting surgeons impressed by our method of anesthesia asked to have their anesthetists trained by us or to have a nurse-anesthetist whom we had trained. Before we knew it, Lakeside had inaugurated its School of Anesthesia.[17]

Crile and Hodgins were justly proud of their Lakeside Hospital of Anesthesia. Hodgins, reflecting in 1941, attributed the "success attending the development of nurse anesthetist service, at this time and in this place" largely to the "*sound* education given by Doctor Crile to the nurse anesthetists into whose hands he had entrusted this work." The school had "from its inception held a high place as an organized center for teaching anesthesiology, contributing much to the education of nurse anesthetists, and furthering, through the work of its graduates, the progress and efficiency of anesthesia service throughout this country."[18] Its beneficial influences were further spread as other schools modeled after it were founded around the country. In 1948, the American Association of Nurse Anesthetists presented its Award of Appreciation, posthumously, to Dr. George Crile. The Association President, Lucy E. Richards, paid homage to his role in supporting the profession, and noted in particular his contribution to education excellence:

Living memorials to him are the 54 formal schools for the training of nurse anesthetists in registered hospitals in this country. Because of his vision and his confidence, the anesthesia service in over 75 per cent of the nation's registered hospitals is being conducted by nurse anesthetists educated in schools patterned after the one of which he was the founder.[19]

Both Crile and Hodgins believed their school to be the first "in the world."[20] Hodgins, who felt herself on firm "historical ground," believed that "This school, by reason of its organizational form; teaching faculty; adequate educational requirements for entrance; defined course of instruction, and awarding of a certificate upon satisfactory completion of the prescribed course, is set apart as a *school* of anesthesia, and differentiated from other and possibly earlier centers of instruction—*none* of which, so far as I can learn, were designated as, or fulfilled the distinct function of such a school per se."[21] But within a few years of Hodgins's death, Thatcher documented the existence of four other hospital "true postgraduate courses in anesthesia" prior to World War I: St. Vincent's Hospital, Portland, Oregon (1909); St. John's Hospital, Springfield, Illinois (1912): the New York Post-Graduate Hospital, New York City (1912); and the Long Island College Hospital, Brooklyn (1914).[22]

Agnes McGee, a 1907 graduate of St. Joseph's Hospital School of Nursing, Chicago, established the course at St. Vincent's Hospital after returning from study in Heidelberg, Germany, where she prepared to be a surgical supervisor and learned anesthesia. Her program "lasted six months and included instruction in anatomy, the physiology of the respiratory tract and the pharmacology of the anesthetic drugs, as well as training in the administration of the then commonly used anesthetic agents."[23] McGee was given the American Association of Nurse Anesthetists' "Award of Appreciation" in 1953. The Award to the Hospital Sisters of the Third Order of St. Francis for their pioneering program at St. John's Hospital has already been noted.

The anesthesia course for graduate nurses at the New York Post-Graduate Hospital lasted six months. "Each student administered anesthesia for 400 cases, attended heart clinics and lectures by physicians and did experimental work with cadavers, which included the passing of laryngeal tubes."[24] At the Long Island College Hospital, the course was also six months long, with lectures delivered by a visiting physician anesthetist.

Just as the practice of using trained nurse anesthetists was spreading, so, too, the establishment of formal educational programs was replacing the practice of nurses and graduate physicians learning anesthesia as visitors to hospitals. World War I, however, delayed further development of some educational programs—including Hodgins's own.

Nurse Anesthetist Service in the Great War

As Crile recalled, "Then came the First World War and the service of the Lakeside Unit at the American Ambulance at Neuilly in 1914. The implication of that was enormous." He added, "We literally introduced gas-oxygen anesthesia into war surgery and into England and France."[25]

Hodgins, who accompanied Crile, recorded the significance for nurse anesthetists:

The unit . . . in [the] charge of Dr. Crile, left in December, 1914, for service in the American Ambulance Hospital, Neuilly, Paris,

France. Attached to this unit were three anesthetists—the writer and two members of her staff. The assignment of this anesthesia unit was to introduce gas-oxygen in war surgery, from that base hospital. The fortunate result was that of being able to successfully accomplish this assignment both on this special unit, and later, on the French surgical division of the American Ambulance Hospital. Thus, nurse anesthetists were certainly among the first, if not the first, from this country in service during the war of 1914. Later, when America entered the war, this service was greatly multiplied and nurse anesthetists from all over the country were sent to France to serve in base hospitals as anesthetists—and a very excellent record they made.[26]

Crile returned to the United States within two months, presenting a plan to the Surgeon-General to create hospital units for service abroad composed of doctors, nurses, and anesthetists. His plan was adopted early in 1915, and leading hospital centers around the country organized units.

Crile saw that "perhaps the prime outstanding problem [on the front] was that of shock and exhaustion."[27] Lakeside's nitrous oxide—oxygen anesthesia was therefore especially appropriate, and Crile noted that "Sir Anthony Bowlby, the Chief Medical Advisor of the British Expeditionary Forces, after observing the comparative effects of ether and of nitrous oxide anesthesia in thousands of operations, advised the adoption of nitrous oxide as the anesthetic of choice in the British hospitals. This anesthetic was already the anesthetic of choice in the American Army, and was later adopted by the French."[28] Unfortunately, there remained a problem of supplying nitrous oxide to the front. Dr. Arthur E. Guedel related that "nitrous oxide here is almost out of the question. I understand Major Crile brought a lot of it over for the Lakeside Unit, but I do not know of any other available source here at our part of the front. A number of units have gas apparatus, but at present *nothing to use in them*."[29] The ingenious and determined Crile, however, succeeded in getting the American Red Cross to buy a plant for manufacturing nitrous oxide—dissembling, shipping, and then reassembling it in France. Crile reported that "it had a capacity of 125,000 gallons per eight-hour operations and was the largest in the world at the time of its construction. It was completed, tested, approved, and shipped from Cleveland early in January, 1918." He added that it was also lost for a time in transit, and only became operational later that summer.[30]

Hodgins stayed on in France after Crile left. There had been requests for her to train others in nitrous oxide—oxygen anesthesia, among them "Berkeley George Moynihan's anesthetist, an American nurse—a Miss Cotton who carried on the work when Agatha Hodgins returned to Cleveland in 1915—two groups of English nurses leaving for posts near the front lines, and several Frenchmen."[31] Then, when the Lakeside Unit was replaced by the Harvard Unit, Dr. Harvey Cushing requested that she stay on, and continue to teach until his new unit was well established.

Hodgins returned to Cleveland to resume work on the Lakeside School of Anesthesia. Its first class graduated in 1916, and included six physicians, two dentists, and eleven nurses. When war was declared by the United States on April 6, 1917, the Lakeside Hospital Unit, designated as "Base Hospital No. 4," was mobilized. This time, however, Hodgins did not accompany Crile. She chose to remain as director of the school, training nurse anesthetists for military service.

Hodgins's successor as Chief Anesthetist of the Lakeside Unit was Mary J. Roche-Stevenson. Other members of the anesthesia team included another nurse anesthetist, Miss Cunningham, and a dentist, Dr. Sykes. Orderlies of the unit were volunteer enlisted men, most of whom were students at Western Reserve University. In recognition of Crile's plan for hospital units, the Lakeside group was accorded the honor of being the first military unit to leave the United States for overseas duty. They left Cleveland on May 6, 1917.

Mary J. Roche-Stevenson published a memoir of her two-year experience in May, 1942—in the midst of another world war. Her graphic description of the heroic service performed by nurse anesthetists foreshadowed that of Patricia L. Walsh in her fictionalized memoir of Vietnam, *Forever Sad the Hearts*. But this was World War I, the first time the army and navy trained nurses as anesthetists for war service, where they "uniquely contributed to battlefield medicine" by "providing much of the anesthesia administered near the front as well as in base hospitals."[32] Roche-Stevenson recalled:

> Work at a Casualty Clearing Station [C.C.S.] came in waves after major battles, with intervals between of very little to do. This was the season of the long and bloody struggle for Passchendaele. Barrages of gun fire would rock the sector for days, then convoys of wounded would begin to arrive by ambulance. Night and day this ceaseless stream kept coming on. Walking wounded were taken care of in a special tent and evacuated immediately by hospital train.
>
> In a receiving tent, the stretcher cases were assembled, stripped of their clothing and dressed in clean, new pajamas. The seriously wounded, especially the ones in severe shock, were taken to a special ward, given blood transfusions and other treatments in preparation for surgery later. From the receiving tent, the wounded were brought to the surgery, put on the operating tables stretcher

and all, given an anesthetic, operated upon, picked up on their stretcher, and loaded on hospital trains for evacuation to base hospitals.

Surgery huts each had about eight operating tables, arranged length-wise, four on each side of the hut. Shelves ran along the walls which served as tables for instruments, sterile dressings, et cetera. Each operating team worked as a unit, was responsible for its equipment, and alternated on day and night shifts.

Ether and chloroform were the anesthetics used by the British. We had brought a supply of anesthetic gases along with us from our base and one gas machine (quite a curiosity over there at that time). On one memorable occasion, when overtaken with an inundation of wounded, with Dr. [William E.] Lower as surgeon, I gave forty nitrous oxide—oxygen anesthesias in a twenty-four hour stretch of duty. For that record, we gathered a bit of fame for ourselves and gas anesthesia.

Fatigue, overwhelming and profound, was the anesthetist's ally here in this front line area. After extensive battles, the wounded arrived in a state of utter exhaustion. Most of them were in a deep sleep when carried into the surgery; many did not even react when ether was administered. Others would be in a state of high excitement, difficult to control.

Surgery was of all types, with many shattered limbs. All one's attention had to be focused on caring for the wounded and not on the shocking sights encountered. All the wounded had been given antitetanic vaccine at the field hospitals, and the shattered limbs had been put in Thomas splints for transportation to the C.C.S. Tags, on a cord around the soldier's neck, showed the man's name and regiment, as well as vaccines and drugs which had been administered at the field hospital. No surgery was attempted at these field hospitals; first aid only was given. Wounded men who had been lying in shell holes for days in inaccessible areas, were a pathetic sight. They had been without food and often without water, and their wounds were frequently a mass of maggots. While not pretty to look at, these industrious little worms proved themselves a formidable foe to the spread of infection.

During the summer of 1917 the deliberate bombing of hospitals took place. Previously all combatants had left hospital areas unmolested. After this time bombing raids were a nightly occurrence when weather permitted. Surgery huts were blacked out with blankets at sundown, and operating teams on duty remained at their posts regardless of bombing raids. Frequently the lighting system was put out of commission during a raid and we carried on with flashlights. Our C.C.S. had several direct hits during that summer and fall, with casualties among our associates. A soldier learns to accept death as casually as he does life, and necessarily becomes, for the time, a fatalist. To quote the British Tommie, "If it has your number, sister, it gets you," a comforting philosophy under duress.

Summer rains in this sector were torrential at times. The C.C.S. was located in the midst of a Belgian hop field and mud was overwhelming. Duck boards throughout the camp provided side-walk facilities. Here history was lived and the pace was fast. Life was thrilling, shocking—an experience never to be forgotten.[33]

Roche-Stevenson contacted facial erysipelas, and had to spend several weeks in a British isolation hospital. She then returned to Rouen, where the waves of casualties continued:

Very shortly, due to great advances made by the enemy, we were virtually a front line hospital. The enemy was at Amiens, uncomfortably close. The same ceaseless tide of wounded ebbed and flowed, and the wounded were cared for and evacuated to England as rapidly as possible. Always the military hospitals must be kept cleared for the next wave of wounded.[34]

Sophie Gran Winton (1887–1989), a graduate of Swedish Hospital, Minneapolis, trained as an anesthetist at the urging of hospital administrator Gustaf W. Olson. She already had five years anesthesia experience and a record of more than ten thousand cases without a fatality when she joined the Army Nursing Corps (then part of the Red Cross) because "it was the patriotic thing to do."[35] Winton and nine other nurses from Minneapolis Hospital Unit No. 26 were assigned to Mobil Hospital No. 1 in the Chateau-Thierry area in France with the pioneering physician anesthetist James T. Gwathmey. She later reported to her former mentor, Olson, that she

gave anesthetics from the first of June [1918] to November after the Armistice. How many anesthetics I gave during the World War I cannot determine, except that when the big drives were on, lasting from a week to ten days, I averaged twenty-five to thirty a day. The first three months I gave chloroform entirely, after which a ruling came that we were to use ether because there had been too many deaths from chloroform in inexperienced hands. Many a night I had to pour ether or chloroform on my finger to determine the amount I was giving, because we had no lights except the surgeon had a searchlight for his work, so the only sign I had to go by was respiration.[36]

Elsewhere she recalled that "during the drives, patients came in so fast that all the surgeons could do was to remove bullets and shrapnel, stop hemorrhages and put iodoform packs in the wound and bandage it. As soon as they were through operating on one patient, I would have to have the next patient anesthetized."[37] She frequently gave anesthesia as shells fell close to the hospital. All the nurses in Winton's unit were awarded the Croix de Guerre. She herself was also awarded six overseas service bars as well as honors from the Overseas Nurses Association, the American Legion, and the Veterans of Foreign Wars. (It is important to note that Winton and her fellow nurses who served in this war, though serving in military organizations, came under the auspices of the Red Cross. They did not receive full military rank, nor the pay and allowances equal to male military personnel. Nor did they receive veterans' compensation.)

There was also Anne Penland, the only anesthetist with the New York Presbyterian Hospital Unit (Base Hospital No. 2), and the first official nurse anesthetist on the British Front. In her diary she described the bombing of casualty clearing stations:

> We saw things, heard things, and went through them, but they were not such things as anybody but the Germans might have termed warfare. Imagine deliberately bombing a camp of wounded, and I don't mean one camp but as many as they could locate. Miss [Beatrice] MacDonald's camp was the first one and it came like a bolt from the heavens; of course, before this nobody had paid a great deal of attention to the Boche planes going over us, as we foolishly gave them credit for letting us alone and attacking soldiers' camps around us. These three camps were attacked or bombed three nights in succession, and you have heard how, fortunately, Major [William] Darrach was not in his tent, as it was blown to bits.[38]

Unfortunately, nurse MacDonald lost an eye from a shrapnel wound.

Penland's expertise in anesthesia contributed to the British decision to train their own nurses in the work; she was later decorated by the British government. This change in British policy is significant, indicating another instance of the influence of America's nurse anesthetists. As the history of the Pennsylvania Hospital Unit (Base Hospital No. 10) recorded: "Throughout the British Army anesthetics had hitherto only been administered by doctors and when shortly after our arrival our women began their work they were greatly astonished. The skill and care which was displayed soon caused their amazement to yield to admiration. The idea was soon adopted by the British authorities, and in the early spring of 1918 classes were formed of British nurses who received instruction at our hospital and at several others, and before the end of the war a number of British nursing sisters were performing the duties in various hospitals throughout the BEF."[39]

Years later, Dr. George Crile would observe that "if the Great War had gone on another year, the British army would have adopted the nurse anesthetists right in the middle of the war."[40] But, as Daryl Pearce has ably shown in her study of the professional anesthetist in Britain, a British nurse anesthetist "might (barely) be acceptable in times of war but definitely not in peacetime."[41] Though the Royal College of Nursing took the position in 1919 that the British nurses should be given "a chance for success" in anesthesia,[42] the field had from the beginning remained within the province of the British physician. Though the administration of anesthetics in Britain depended heavily on the "occasional" physician anesthetist, and though—just as in the United States—it would be a struggle to secure recognition of anesthesia as a full medical specialty, the British physician was not disposed to surrender ground to the nurse "technician"[43]—a term of derogation that would figure significantly in the debate within the United States.

Anesthesia as Women's Work

While the American nurse anesthetists were risking their lives at the front in volunteer service, establishing an enviable record and winning the admiration of the most celebrated surgeons and medical practitioners in the western world, other voices were being raised at home. There was an awareness that nurses were solidifying their position in the field.

At the thirty-seventh annual meeting of the South Dakota State Medical Association at Mitchell, South Dakota, in May, 1918, Dr. Robert Emmett Farr, the Minneapolis surgeon (mentioned earlier in connection with his coinage of the term "psycho-anesthetist" to describe the contribution of the nurse anesthetist to his successful use of local anesthesia in pediatric surgery), lamented in a discussion on professional anesthetists: "But we are up against this proposition. The war is going to have this influence. We are not going to have physicians enough to give anesthetics, and the nurses are being worked in to give anesthetics. And when the war is over they are coming back here, and they are going to continue to do it; and we are up against that sort of thing."[44]

It will be recalled that early discussion on the need for professional anesthetists returned again and again to the economic factor: without the prospect of attractive and competitive remuneration, talented physicians and interns had no incentive to concentrate on the giving of anesthetics. Nor was there appeal in accepting a subservient, secondary role: "Anaesthesia was born a slave; and she has ever remained the faithful handmaid of her master Surgery," observed the foremost British anesthetist, Dr. Frederic W. Hewitt, in 1896.[45] What was required were people who would:

(1) be satisfied with the subordinate role that the work required,
(2) make anesthesia their one absorbing interest,
(3) not look on the situation of anesthetist as one that put them in a position to watch and learn from the surgeon's technic,
(4) accept comparatively low pay and
(5) have the natural aptitude and intelligence to develop a high level of skill in providing the smooth anesthesia and relaxation that the surgeon demanded.[46]

Not surprisingly, surgeons found these qualities, as the imagery suggests, in women. As hospital administrator Olson reminded his nurse anesthetist audience in 1940, American women were *recruited* into anesthesia, a field "shunned"[47] by physicians: "A fact which should never be lost sight of by doctors, lawmakers, the laity, or the nurses themselves is, that nurses were *drafted* to give anesthetics under the instruction and supervision of surgeons, after it had been found that medical graduates were often inept and lacking the deftness and tender touch which patients required for a successful anesthetic, or they were too much interested in the operator's procedure and therefore failed to give a satisfactory performance as anesthetists."[48] Olson noted that surgeons had learned to have confidence in trained nurses from other demonstrations of not only their competence and reliability, but of their *supportiveness*. His comments here appealed to and glorified the nurse's role of "physician's hand" and helpmate to the surgeon "Captain of the Ship"—an unappealing role for the male physician: "Surgeons knew that nurses were trained to carry out doctors' orders promptly, accurately and faithfully. They observed at every operation how the competent surgical nurse anticipated every requirement to an even greater degree than the medical graduate assistant. They knew that they could depend upon the nurses in the wards to carry out the difficult as well as the simpler orders for the postoperative care of even their most serious cases. They had learned to cast worry aside when there was a competent nurse at the bedside." Olson concluded that *"It was only natural,* then, that the surgeon should turn to the graduate nurse when he wanted a thoroughly trustworthy assistant to carry out his orders for the administration of surgical anesthesia."[49] (emphasis added)

"It was only natural." What was fundamentally an *economic* issue resolved by utilizing talented, trained women, frequently was veiled, unconsciously and/or consciously, in a romantic aura praising the "natural" appropriateness of women as anesthetists, labeling their expertise and concern for patients as uniquely "feminine." Crile, we have seen, called it "finesse," and declared, "I do not think a man can ever have the finesse in the administration of an anesthetic that a woman has."[50] He continued:

> I can illustrate this no better than by citing the finesse of Miss [Lou] Adams in dealing with a little patient two or three years old who had an exophthalmic goiter, and was a very desperate risk. Miss Adams took two or three weeks' time to become acquainted with that little child, to play with the child, give it toys and have it understand the gas machine until finally she had the child's complete confidence without any struggle on the part of the child. That is symbolic of what I meant when I referred to the finesse of the nurse anesthetist as compared with that of the intern. It represents a contribution that I do not believe can ever be equalled among doctors. (1936)[51]

Another surgeon, Philemon E. Truesdale, provided this reasoning:

> Why should not a nurse be a good anesthetist, if she is properly trained by temperament and by intellect? Because she has certain qualities that a man does not possess, and just as soon as the patient lies down to take his ether, if he is a man he gives up to the nurse, but if a man is going to administer that ether the feeling of resistance and fight is in him, and it stays in him until somebody puts their knee on his chest and he is overcome. (1913)[52]

And from surgeon Morton J. Tendler:

> The only treatment which stands out, during spinal anesthesia, is the dulcet note of a musical feminine voice pouring out sweet words of comfort into the anxious brain of a husky man or a pretty miss. It is just too difficult to envision a fat, bald-headed man, with horn-rimmed glasses, pouring sweet nothings into one's ear at any time— let alone at such a crisis in one's life. (1939)[53]

The sex-role metaphor is developed in detail by Hewitt, quoted briefly above. The entire conceit merits attention:

> Anaesthesia was born a slave; and she has ever remained the faithful handmaid of her master Surgery. The gigantic work which

has been and is still being accomplished by the latter would never have been possible without the aid of the former. By the assistance which Anaesthesia has rendered, countless advances and developments in surgical science have resulted. Moreover, Anaesthesia has calmed the public mind. In past years the services of her master were only requisitioned as a last resource; they are now as often invoked in doubtful or obscure cases, and in those in which inconvenience rather than actual suffering has to be remedied. By her influence, too, the very nature and disposition of her master have been modified and softened. The constant infliction of pain to which he had grown accustomed tended to dull the edges of natural sympathy, and to bring about in him an apparent if not a true heartlessness of demeanour and disposition. All this has been changed by Anaesthesia. There is nothing, indeed, to prevent the surgeon of to-day from practising his calling with that gentleness of manner and kindliness of purpose which have hitherto been regarded as belonging more particularly to the physician. (1896)[54]

If anesthesia is the gentling handmaid of surgery, then it is not surprising that women were chosen for the role. In anesthesia, patriarchal values—the assumption that sex differences imply a "natural" separation of activities and a "natural" dominance of male over female—and economics meshed. Nor is it surprising that women, sharing the same cultural bias, accepted the reasoning. As late as 1953, nurse anesthetist historian Thatcher wrote, "Like the woman teacher, the woman nurse anesthetist not only was called into service by desperate need but also brought to her work a natural aptitude that made her superior to the man."[55] Ironically, the gender argument gave women access to a new field of endeavor while at the same time undercutting the significance of their achievement.

It was not only the female nurse who was given a new opportunity. As Dr. Selma H. Calmes has documented in her valuable historical studies, the same factors that opened anesthesia practice to nurses functioned to open the field to female physicians. The low pay and status that made anesthesia an unattractive specialty for the male physician offered an accepted area of practice for the female physician. Faced with obstacles in gaining acceptance in many other areas of medicine, women physicians were seen by many as a desirable presence in anesthesia because they combined the "naturally" appropriate female traits of submissiveness and physical attractiveness with medical knowledge. Also, because of the limited career choices available to them, it was possible to recruit the most talented of women. As Dr. Albert J. Ochsner (who also supported nurse anesthetists) wrote in the 1920 edition of his surgery text: "The best anesthesias are conducted by women at the present time, because it is possible to select women with the highest degree of intelligence and judgement for this work, while medical men possessing these qualities can almost never be induced to elect anesthesia as a specialty."[56] Dr. Arthur Dean Bevan, sharing the belief that "women . . . make the best anesthetists,"[57] recommended that "the talented nurse, who desires to become an anesthetist, study medicine and become licensed."[58]

Calmes has also documented the significant role women physicians played in professional medical anesthesia associations in the years 1920–1950. As men entered the medical specialty in greater numbers, however, the women had a less prominent role.[59]

There is evidence that women physicians tried to distance themselves from the other women in anesthesia, the nurse anesthetists. The professional bond with other physicians would be stronger than the gender bond with other women. Thus, in a paper read before the Medical Society of the State of California in 1920, "The Present Status of Anesthesiology and the Anesthetist," Dr. Eleanor Seymour began by recalling the Genesis story of the "first anesthesia": "The Lord caused a deep sleep to fall upon Adam and he slept, and He took one of his ribs and closed up the flesh instead thereof." She then ironically observed:

> It is cause for regret that there is no detailed account of the induction and maintenance of this first anesthetic but it is evident that the administration was considered of such importance as not to be entrusted even to the Angel Gabriel,—much less an angelic nurse,—and of Adam's safe and satisfactory recovery there is abundant record.[60]

Seymour would become president of the Associated Anesthetists of the United States and Canada in 1923.

Dr. Mary Botsford—whom Calmes identifies as probably the first woman physician anesthetist—was a prominent and charismatic figure who dominated West Coast anesthesia for twenty years. Working at The Children's Hospital of San Francisco, Botsford trained at least forty-six women medical graduates in the specialty of anesthesia. It seems not unlikely that her influence played a part in the 1921 action of a female intern in a San Francisco hospital. Refusing to take instruction in anesthesia from a nurse, the woman was expelled for insubordination. She appealed to the County Medical Society and was sustained in her position. The intern was reinstated and the nurse instructor was dropped.[61]

Dr. Virginia Apgar (famous for creation of the Apgar Score) began her medical career in anesthesia. Interestingly, her initial instruction in anesthesia was at the hands of nurse anesthetist Anne Penland, who returned to Presbyterian Hospital after World War I, and was its chief anesthetist for twenty years.[62] After further study with Dr. Ralph M. Waters and Dr. Emery A. Rovenstine, Apgar began the Division of Anesthesia at Columbia-Presbyterian Medical Center in 1937. Writing to Waters, seeking his help in finding residents for her new training program, she requested, "no women yet."[63] Calmes points out that, though it was not uncommon for the first residents in such training programs to be female, Apgar's first three were male.[64]

Though not a physician, Laurette McMechan shared the work and passionate conviction of her husband. Dr. Frank McMechan was a pioneering leader in the professional organization of physician anesthesia and probably the most virulent of the opponents to nurse anesthetists. The journal *Anesthesiology*, launched in 1940 by the physician group, the American Society of Anesthesiologists, owes its existence in part to the refusal of the widowed Laurette to compromise the stance she had taken with her husband: "There was no place in organized anesthesia for nurse anesthetists and they wanted no part of any organization that either tolerated or endorsed (as did the A.M.A.) nurse anesthetists."[65] She would not permit the McMechan journal, *Current Researches in Anesthesia and Analgesia,* to become associated with a less "orthodox" group. This was then a factor in the ASA decision to proceed with the new publication.

If the women in medical anesthesia felt the need to distance themselves from other women in anesthesia—the nurse anesthetists who, as nurses, occupied a lower place in the professional hierarchy—the problem for the male physicians in anesthesia was even greater. Seeking to gain status for anesthesia as a medical specialty, with its accompanying privileges and money, they had, in the words of Rosemary Stevens, "to contend with the female image."[66] It is not surprising, then, that the Waters-Rovenstine correspondence manifested that "both had an antipathy toward women in medicine, particularly women in anesthesia."[67] In addition, Calmes notes that, "Guedel wrote to Waters in 1931, 'However I do not believe in women doctors.' Waters responded, 'You have nothing on me in your attitude towards that.' Guedel answered later, 'I still feel as usual about women anesthetists.'"[68] To move anesthesia from "handmaid" status, the female image had to be eradicated. To gain recognition for anesthesia as a science, the notion that success was due to "nature" or "art" had to be overcome. To make anesthesia a respectable field for the physician, the contributions of the nurse had to be ignored or denied or denigrated. Some, in their zeal to establish a late claim that anesthesia was the exclusive domain of the physician, declared nurse anesthetists an "abuse" or an "evil" to be outlawed by the courts.

·3·

A Very Personal Property Right

In their 1918 discussion, Dr. Robert E. Farr and his colleagues reflected the continuing frustration that economics made anesthesia unattractive to physician specialists. There was also voiced the frustration that nurses were establishing themselves in the field and adding a competitive dimension to the already difficult economic situation.

The paper occasioning the discussion is of particular importance because it was delivered by Dr. Ralph M. Waters, then specializing in anesthesia in Sioux City, Iowa. A graduate of Western Reserve University, he cited elsewhere three reasons for his interest in anesthesia:

> First, the results of anesthesia which I observed were variable and offered something of a challenge. Second, extra-curricular experience in the administration of anesthetics while a student in Cleveland, together with occasional opportunities to observe the use of nitrous oxide by the extremely skillful dentist, Charles K. Teter, had developed in me an unusual interest in the subject. And lastly, one of the more "surgical" surgeons returned from an eastern trip in 1913 with a nitrous oxide apparatus (the first in Sioux City) the use of which he offered to me in other cases if I would anesthetize his patients.[1]

In 1927 Waters would join the faculty of the new medical school of the University of Wisconsin, and come to be known as the "Father of Academic Anesthesia." A charismatic pioneer of physician anesthesia, Waters vigorously opposed nurse anesthetists. (It is, therefore, especially ironic that both Waters and Hodgins's mentor, Crile, were influenced by the Cleveland dentist, Dr. Teter and his work with nitrous oxide.) Waters's presentation here is permeated with his frustration over the medical profession's lack of interest in anesthesia.

He begins with the observation: "I hear that some surgeon in this state is using *a nurse or an office girl—I'm not sure which*—to administer anesthetics to his patients. Do you know why? The only honorable reason he could give is because he believes that she can give an anesthetic better than any practitioner of medicine available in his community. Surgeons with this handicap can be found in many communities in the United States today."[2] (emphasis added) To help correct this situation, Waters appeals to the "physicians (both women and men) in every town who occasionally give anesthetics to wake up, get busy, and make anesthesia a part or all of your business." He assures them that they "will be surprised at the amount of reading along this line that you can find," and that "anesthesia is a science worth while." *So* worthwhile, that "*It is not a nurse's job which you must be ashamed to have to perform—to feel concerning it as you would at being caught giving a soapsuds enema.* It is a physician's job; an art, if you please, just as much as surgery is an art, and requires training, reading, and work to do it well." (emphasis added) These comments are perhaps the most telling glimpse into the dilemma of a physician moving into a field associated with nursing.[3]

Waters assures his physician audience that not only is anesthesia "more interesting than the giving of a soapsuds enema," it is also more interesting than "watching of the drops as they fall from a Squibb's ¼-lb. can onto a gauze mask"—a reference to the open-drop method nurses had raised to a subtle art and which was the subject of the British physician anesthetist discussion above.

There is a contradiction in Waters's argument. On the one hand he urges physicians to involve themselves more deeply than at present, even if only on a part-time basis: "This does not mean, necessarily, an exclusive specialty. *Every man must have a hobby.*" (emphasis added) Yet, he also cautions that the technic of nitrous oxide and oxygen anesthesia "is of such a fine nature that you have to keep at it every day and study it right along in order to keep up." His comments reflect the low status of nursing: what might be a suitable hobby for a physician is not a suitable career for a nurse.

Waters's discussion of advances in nitrous oxide and oxygen anesthesia does allude to Crile: "There is a development the world over in the administration of anesthetics and in nitrous oxide and oxygen, particularly because that is receiving more attention from men who have gone into the subject in detail, because it seems to be the nearest to the ideal." But Waters makes no mention of Crile's choice of a nurse for his anesthetist, nor to his support of a school to train nurse anesthetists. Likewise, his colleague Dr. C. E. McCauley takes note of the support of the Mayo surgeons for their nurse anesthetists, but does not acknowledge their accomplishments:

Up in this Northwestern country, particularly, we have gotten into pretty bad habits. I do not like to call names, but I think the Rochester Clinic has been responsible for this. They make the claim down there that a nurse makes a better anesthetist (I have heard Dr. W. W. Mayo say this) than the average doctor.[4]

This refusal to acknowledge publicly any meaningful contribution by pioneering nurse anesthetists will be repeated by physician-anesthetist authors over the years, with the result of a denial to nurse anesthetists of a just place in the literature of the field. It results in an historical "invisibility" which, as women—*and* nurses—they share with other lower-status groups as well as racial and ethnic minorities.

Another theme of these discussants is that of the economic obstacles to physician anesthesia and the competition that nurses bring to the field: "The reason we have not better men or a larger number of good men giving general anesthetics, is that we do not see that they are properly paid." Dr. McCauley elaborates:

I think the main reason that we are having nurses give anesthetics, at least up in this country, is the question of money. In most of the towns you will find some men who are good anesthetists. We have one or two in our city who are good anesthetists; but we have a fixed fee for a great deal of our work. You will find that the average fee for small work, such as tonsils, is $25, $35, or $50. The average fee for major operations runs between $100 and $200. Suppose I do twenty-five operations a month. It would cost me $10 for the majors and $5 for the minors on an average where they are done under an anesthetic. I am going to pay out anywhere from one hundred to one hundred and fifty dollars a month for anesthesia, and if I can hire a girl who will keep my instruments clean, and who will do my office work, etc., I can get her for about sixty-odd dollars a month, and I am making from one to two hundred dollars a month clear on that alone.

As nurses were building their reputation, actions were being taken to legislate them out of existence. Just as the discussion above made no distinction between competent and incompetent nurse anesthetists, so too the legal efforts were directed against *all* nurse anesthetists. But then it probably had to be so. It was the demonstrated competency that created the competition. As Dr. George W. Crile later observed, "If it had happened that the nurse anesthetist had accidents that could have been avoided, if the nurse anesthetist had not been steadfast in the midst of trouble, if she would not stay at her post in times of great crisis or if she could not be depended upon, that would have been an entirely different matter."[5]

Organized Anti-Nurse Anesthetist Activity

The center of *organized* anti-nurse anesthetist activity rested in Dr. Francis Hoeffer McMechan, a native of Cincinnati. A third-generation physician, McMechan came to medicine after an undergraduate career focused on oratory, debating, and dramatics, and three years' employment on the *Cincinnati Post.* "About the time he was beginning to consider himself a newspaperman, his father said: 'Frank, I think you have fooled around enough now, and it is time you went to medical school'."[6] McMechan took a special interest in anesthesia, though, he said, "In 1903, I found the profession rather amazed that a young doctor could fool away his time at anything so inconsequential as putting patients to sleep."[7] His general practice, with its growing emphasis on anesthesia, was halted when, around 1911, he developed arthritis and was confined to a wheelchair for the rest of his life. Unable to practice medicine, and faced with financial hardship, McMechan found redirection, utilizing his considerable skills in theater and journalism. "At this time, he became concerned about better organization of the field of anesthesia, and he felt that his confinement would give him time to be productive in this regard."[8]

One focus of McMechan's work would be in publishing. He later recalled: "In the meantime, in seeking a new outlet for my shut-in limitations, it occurred to me that a journal on anesthesia would be greatly needed, not only to further the organization of the specialty, but more especially to broadcast its literature."[9] Severely crippled, McMechan was assisted and supported by his wife, Laurette, who assumed an ever-increasing role in his work. They also shared the intractable belief, alluded to above, that there was no place in anesthesia for the nurse.

This conviction that anesthesia belonged to physicians was expanded in his 1935 address to the Council on Medical Education and Licensure of the American Medical Association, "Should the Radiologist, the Pathologist, and the Anesthetist be Licensed to Practice Medicine?" McMechan argued: "The code of medical ethics has come to me, representing the third generation of Ohio doctors in my family, as a sacred heritage; as one of the group of doctors to pass the first Ohio State Medical Board examination, my license to practice has always meant *a very personal property right* to me, and an experience of 30 years in anesthesia has convinced me that anesthesia must be limited to licensed and qualified physicians to achieve its destiny—the conquest of human pain."[10] (emphasis added) After establishing his property rights, McMechan continued by presenting his brief history of anesthesia: "Anesthesia was the gift of pioneer doctors and dentists to suffering humanity, and *every significant advance in its science and practice has been contributed by doctors, dentists and research workers of similar standing. In contrast, technicians have added nothing of any consequence.*"[11] (emphasis added) As in the 1918 physician discussion, there is again a denial of *any* contribution on the part of nurse anesthetists. Nor will McMechan even utter their name, only the denigrating label, "technicians."

The influence of the McMechans as a pro-physician, anti-nurse anesthetist force was far-reaching. As Waters noted: "Of the anesthetists who were living between 1912 and 1939, it is doubtful if there was a single one who did not know him personally and count the McMechans his friends. The McMechans made the get-together spirit that lives after him among the anesthetists of the world."[12] It was, in effect, McMechan who welcomed Waters to the specialty.[13]

Beginning in 1911, with the onslaught of his illness, McMechan was a motivating force in the organization of physician anesthesia. Where such organization occurred, legal action against the existence of nurse anesthetists was usually close behind:

In 1911, McMechan helped found the New York Society of Anesthetists, which succeeded the Long Island Society of Anesthetists. A year later in 1912, the New York society petitioned the American Medical Association to create a section on anesthesia at its annual meeting in Atlantic City, but was not successful. However, from this effort, the American Association of Anesthetists, which had held sporadic informal meetings for five or six years, was formally organized at the AMA meeting in Atlantic City, in 1912. This group held their first meeting at the same time as the AMA, in June 1913 in Minneapolis, where McMechan presented a paper on "The Medical-Legal Status of Anesthesia."[14]

In 1915, Dr. McMechan, with Dr. E. I. McKession of Toledo, Ohio, and Dr. William Hamilton Long of Louisville, Kentucky, organized the Interstate Association of Anesthetists, and this became the nucleus for further regional societies in the United States and Canada.[15]

A few manufacturers and McMechan met in the Union Club of Cleveland on December 18, 1919, to discuss the possibilities of an educational campaign, providing a bulletin, and the formation of a formal organization. As a consequence, the National Anesthesia Research Society was founded. . . . *Current Researches in Anesthesia and Analgesia,* [its] publication was born with the first issue appearing in August, 1922.[16]

The early 1920s saw the organization of several regional physician-anesthetist societies, to a great degree a testimony to the McMechans: the Canadian Society of Anaesthetists, 1921; the Pacific Coast Association of Anesthetists, 1922; the Southern Association of Anesthetists, 1922; the Eastern Society of Anesthetists, 1923. In 1926, the Interstate Association of Anesthetists became the Midwestern Association of Anesthetists. The American Association of Anesthetists became the Associated Anesthetists of the United States and Canada. McMechan's own National Anesthesia Research Society became the International Anesthesia Research Society in 1925. During these years, "not only did McMechan direct extensive planning in connection with the organizing and operation of these societies, but he and Mrs. McMechan made many trips each year to attend their meetings."[17] Effective and committed, "with the completion of these organizations, McMechan was realizing his goals. American [physician] anesthesia was being consolidated."[18]

A consideration of the major legal and political actions taken against nurse anesthetists during these years also reveals McMechan's hand. He used the editorial pages of his quarterly *Anesthesia Supplement* of the *American Journal of Surgery* to "make every effort to abolish the evils involved in the administration of anesthetics by non-medical anesthetists,"[19] and recommended legal and political strategies that were, in fact, adopted by his constituency. For example, in April, 1915, he urged that "*hospital trustees should be compelled* to protect the lives of patients entrusted to their care, by having all general anesthetics administered by or under the supervision of staff- or visiting-[medical] anesthetists. In this connection it is imperative that the *Medical Practice Acts of the various States be so amended* as to abolish the present menace of the nurse-anesthetist, and that medical associations should *question the ethical standing of those surgeons* who persist in employing lay-[nurse] anesthetists, in the presence of competent, licensed practitioners, who are ready to undertake the work and shoulder its full responsibilities."[20] (emphasis added)

McMechan attacked explicitly the "economic crime" committed against the medical profession when nurses were employed as anesthetists. For example, in his July, 1915, column, he declared: "The nurse anesthetist must go because she is unlicensed, and because her employment is as much an economic crime against the profession and public as *fee-splitting.*" He then urged the American College of Surgeons, "some of [whose] most prominent members . . . continue the routine employment of unlicensed anesthetists" (i.e., nurse anesthetists), to "take action in this matter" and thereby cease "alienating a certain proportion of licensed practitioners from a legitimate source of financial support."[21]

The repeated public charge was that nurse anesthetists were violating medical practice acts (or, to use McMechan's phrase, infringing on physicians' "very personal property rights"). Actions flowed from the newly organized physician groups. In New York (organized in 1911), "the legality of nurse anesthesia came into question and an opinion was handed down by the counsel for the New York State Medical Society. In 1911, this counsel, James Taylor Lewis, declared that the administration of an anesthetic by a nurse was in violation of the law of the State of New York."[22]

The Challenge to Lakeside Hospital

The following year, action began in Ohio, home both to McMechan and Lakeside Hospital, against its nurse anesthesia program. Crile received a letter from the secretary of the Ohio State Medical Board informing him of its position that no one other than a registered physician could administer an anesthetic. The board also noted that the Attorney General concurred in his opinion.[23] The next step came in 1916, when "the Interstate Association of Anesthetists [organized in 1915], acting through Frank H. McMechan, petitioned the Ohio State Medical Board to take action against Lakeside Hospital 'as the chief source of the nurse-anesthetist abuse.' "[24] The Board's adopted resolution read:

> *Whereas;* it has been charged in a petition, signed by many well-known and reputable physicians, that the law regarding the administration of anesthetics by others than licensed physicians has been systematically violated by Lakeside Hospital, Cleveland, Ohio, and that courses in anesthetics are given nurses in Lakeside Hospital for the purpose and with the intent of violating the above mentioned law, therefore,

> *Be It Resolved,* that until these charges are disproven and such courses, if given, discontinued, that all recognition of the Lakeside Hospital as an acceptable Training School for Nurses be withheld and recognition of its graduates as Registered Nurses shall be denied.[25]

To prevent denial of recognition of its nursing school, Lakeside Hospital discontinued the anesthesia school, as a debate ensued before the medical board. McMechan argued that Ohio "is the pivotal state . . . in the national fight for the *preservation* [sic] of the status of the anesthetist as a [medical] specialist."[26] (emphasis added) Interestingly, Crile, who on other occasions took pride in his leadership role in supporting nurse anesthetists, argued here that Lakeside Hospital was following "the lead . . . taken by many of the large clinics of the country."[27] The hearing resulted in a withdrawal of the edict. The Lakeside school reopened in 1917 with increased applications from 141 nurses and 31 physicians.

When the Interstate Association of Anesthetists initiated its action in Ohio in 1916 it also adopted a resolution to "bring to an end the administration of anesthetics by unlicensed persons in every state in the middle West in which such action can be secured."[28] In fact Kentucky, the home state of one of the founders of the Interstate Association of Anesthetists, Dr. William Hamilton Long, was the site of a simultaneous action.

Frank v. South

The Louisville Society of Anesthetists submitted its resolution that an anesthetic should be administered only by one who had medical knowledge and training to the Attorney General, who gave a supporting opinion. The House of Delegates of the Kentucky State Medical Association subsequently passed a resolution sponsored by its Committee on Medical Ethics calling for an end to the "evil" of nonphysician anesthetists: "In order therefore, to stop this evil now, your Committee recommends that the medical profession of Kentucky request its members not to employ others than qualified physicians as anesthetists except in cases of emergency. In order to make this request urgent and effective, we would suggest that the profession should not refer cases to hospitals where nurses are allowed to give anesthetics, and that hereafter no member who so violates the law and ethics shall be considered in good standing in this Association."[29] Ironically, nurses, who were called into anesthesia because it was a field shunned by physicians, were now to be themselves shunned.

A Louisville surgeon, Dr. Louis Frank, and his anesthetist, Margaret Hatfield, a graduate nurse with special anesthesia training, insisted that the State Board of Health be party to a test court case. The original finding was against Frank and Hatfield. This was appealed, however, and reversed. The opinion by Judge Hurt discussed the significant issues of "property rights" versus public good and the overlapping "provinces" of various healing professions:

> The appellees insist, that, upon the facts agreed upon and the proof on file, that the appellant, Margaret Hatfield, is practicing

medicine within the meaning of the law in this state, while the contrary is the contention of the appellants. The court below held to the view of the appellees and hence this appeal. . . . [These] laws have not been enacted for the peculiar benefit of the members of such professions, further than they are members of the general community, but they have been enacted for the benefit of the people. . . .

While the practice of medicine is one of the most noble and learned professions, it is apparent that such a construction ought not to be given to the statute, which regulates the profession, that the effect of it would be to invade the province of the professions of pharmacy, dentistry or trained nursing, all of which are professions, which relate to the alleviation of the human family of sickness and bodily afflictions, and to make duties belonging to those professions, also "the practice of medicine" within the meaning of the statute. Neither should such a construction be given to it as to deprive the people from all service, which could be rendered to them in sickness and affliction, except gratuitous service, or else by licensed physicians, unless the legislature intended that such should be the result of the enactment of the statute. . . .

We are of the opinion that in the performance of the services by appellant, Hatfield, in the way and under the circumstances as agreed upon, as being the facts in this case, that she is not engaged in the practice of medicine within the meaning of the statute laws upon that subject, and hence the judgment appealed from is reversed and the cause remanded for proceedings consistent with this opinion.[30]

In spite of such failures as the Lakeside Hospital action and *Frank v. South,* McMechan and other physician anesthetists continued their efforts. He reported on some of them in his *Anesthesia Supplement* in October, 1921:

In the present session of the Colorado Legislature a new Medical Practice Act was killed in Committee because it was against public welfare. Some surgeons and nurses were prepared to try and amend this new legislation so as to enable nurses to give anesthetics.

In Ohio, after the bill repealing nurse anesthesia had been passed by an overwhelming vote in the Senate, and had been endorsed by the House of Delegates of the Ohio State Medical Association by a vote of 63 to 10, it was held up in the House until the closing hours of the session. At this time efforts were made to amend it to death, but these were defeated. The floor leader then retired it in favor of tax legislation and just before final adjournment put it to a vote, when not enough legislators were present to pass it. In consequence the bill died with the passing of the session.

The Ohio State Medical Association, however, through its President and Council has settled on a definite policy on anesthesia. . . . Apparently all opposition within the Ohio State Medical Association against repealing nursing anesthesia is centered in Cleveland. . . .

During the final Executive Session of the American Association of Anesthetists [organized in 1912] at the Boston meeting, the following resolutions was [sic] adopted:

"Be It Resolved, That in the future no member of the American Association of Anesthetists shall instruct any undergraduate nurse or orderly in the art of anesthesia, with the intention of granting them a certificate or diploma qualifying them as competent anesthetists.

"Be It Further Resolved, That nothing in this resolution shall effect [sic] the instruction of medical students in regular medical schools or teaching hospitals or the routine teaching of nursing."

During the meeting of the Ontario Medical Association at Niagara Falls, Canada, the draft of a new Medical Practice Act . . . makes anesthesia an inviolable part of the practice of medicine.[31]

In 1946, Waters acknowledged that McMechan's style—and substance—caused conflict within the medical community: "The recognition and advancement of [physician] anesthesia were very dear to his heart. Opposition was frequently encountered. At times he vented his wrath upon surgeons and representatives of our national medical organizations, and many of these returned the compliment, with interest. Such conflicts were unfortunate and valueless. By some they were thought to have obstructed the advancement of the cause which he sought to promote."[32] But, such reservations notwithstanding, Waters considered McMechan to have contributed the most to [physician] anesthesia: "Is not the man who can bring together the knowledge of a specialty that is scattered throughout the world, promote its discussion, inspire further investigation *and cement all the interested individuals together with the common bond of friendship*—is not such a man the greatest benefactor to his specialty?[33] (emphasis added)

Through McMechan's organizing and publishing and through Waters's teaching, these two unquestionably charismatic leaders shaped physician anesthesia in this country. They also left a formidable legacy of anti-nurse anesthetist sentiment.

·4·

A Matter for Felicitation

I said we can get nowhere without an organization. We're in the minority, of course, but we must organize. And so that night started the organization of the Nurse Anesthetists Association.[1]

The year was 1930; the city was Los Angeles; the speaker was Adeline Curtis, a nurse anesthetist who had been fighting the efforts to outlaw nurse anesthetists in California.

Around the same time, Hilda Salomon, at Jewish Hospital in Philadelphia, organized a local group. She recalled thinking that, given the number of nurse anesthetists in the area, it would be beneficial for them to meet to "compare notes and learn" from each other's experience:

I got on the phone and I called the anesthetists at every hospital and sure enough arranged for them to come to the Jewish Hospital for a meeting once every month. Each one of us, there were perhaps about ten or fifteen in the group, would present difficult cases and how we handled these cases. The discussion was open, with no ill feeling, but they criticized, they congratulated, they praised one another and it was a great help. It was an education in itself.[2]

Learning that there had been an earlier state association of nurse anesthetists that had since disbanded, Salomon began expanding her invitations to include other cities.

In the meantime, Agatha Hodgins had organized her Lakeside alumnae into the Alumnae Association of the Lakeside School of Anesthesia in 1923. Three years later, this inactive group was reorganized, but clearly not with a view to remaining a local entity. At the first meeting Hodgins presented her plan for a national organization of nurse anesthetists, and a preliminary constitution and bylaws were written. She would, in fact, see it established in 1931.

During these years, then, various nurse anesthetist professional societies were formed for different reasons, each with different emphases, reflecting the personality and view of its founder. As Emerson observed, an institution is the lengthened shadow of one person. If Curtis was aggressive and Salomon benevolent, Hodgins was visionary. This woman with the "very interesting personality" had years earlier realized that nurse anesthesia was a special field of "endeavor,"[3] requiring special professional recognition and safeguards. She was committed to converting others to her vision, and (not unlike McMechan) was vexed with those slow to share it.

Chief among objects of her impatience was the American Nurses' Association. It resulted in what Ira Gunn, CRNA, later called a "civil war" in nursing.[4]

In 1941 Hodgins related the various occasions of her disappointment with the ANA. The first was in 1909. Hodgins's reflections thirty-two years later were still charged with emotion:

> In 1909 or thereabouts, Florence Henderson, Miss MacGaw's [sic] successor, was invited to give at a biennial convention of the American Association a paper on *ether* versus gas anesthesia, and I, as an exponent of gas-oxygen, was invited to discuss her paper. I regretfully record that while Miss Henderson and myself both regarded our papers, to put it modestly, well above the average, we were evidently quite alone in this opinion, and the appearance of two supposedly famous pioneers caused not a ripple on the surface of that convention, doubtless due to the fact, that accomplishing pioneers, the American Nurses' Association is the ne plus ultra and so although we thought we were good, we were apparently not good enough.[5]

Hodgins then cited another incident, this one in 1921. She had accepted an invitation to present a paper on "Nurse Anesthetist Service" before the Cleveland division of The League of Nursing Education. Hodgins felt that an opportunity to counter anti–nurse anesthetist activity should not be lost.

> In this paper I outlined the arguments advanced by the medical anesthetists against nurse anesthetist service, offering in rebuttal the reasons why this service was valuable and should be supported. While I thought I was a pretty fair advocate, and presented a good case, I was apparently not yet *good enough* for the American Nurses' Association.[6] (original emphasis)

Hodgins, however, did see a connection between her presentation in 1921 and a move in 1930 to organize a group combining nurse anesthetists and office nurses: "The only result of this—if result it can be called—was a much later invitation from a group of nurse anesthetists, evidently influenced by a group within the American Nurses' Association, to organize as a section in that association 'Office Nurses and Nurse Anesthetists.' "[7] It was Anne E. Beddow, of Alabama, who lead the effort to organize a section combining these groups. Hodgins's perception notwithstanding, it would have been a logical direction to a Southern nurse because, as Thatcher pointed out, these duties were most commonly combined in that region. The resolution was presented at the 1930 biennial meeting of the American Nurses' Association in Milwaukee. Hodgins related that "knowledge of the possibility of this unfortunate development" led her to her delivering a paper at the meeting. According to her subsequent self-evaluation of that presentation:

This paper did, I sincerely believe, help to make nurse anesthetists there present realize the importance of nurse anesthetist service as a separate division of hospital service—not a section of nursing or related in any sense (except that office nurses sometimes are called upon to administer anesthetics) to this division of nursing.[8]

The resolution was revised, calling for further discussion in state and other local ANA meetings; it subsequently died.

After the Milwaukee meeting, Hodgins moved quickly to develop a national organization. In May 1931 she invited Lakeside alumnae as well as other nurse anesthetists around the country (including, for example, Hilda Salomon) to "attend a meeting for the purpose of considering the organization of the nurse anesthetist group."[9] In spite of her strongly declared conviction that nurse anesthesia service be a separate hospital service and not part of its nursing service, she would seek its affiliation with the American Nurses' Association.

Forty nurse anesthetists from twelve states met in a classroom at Western Reserve University on June 17, 1931. The minutes record:

Persuant [sic] to a call issued by Miss Agatha C. Hodgins for the purpose of establishing an International Association of Nurse Anesthetists, a mass meeting was held Wednesday June 17 in the class room of the Department of Anesthesia, University-Lakeside Hospital in Cleveland, Ohio at 2:30 P.M.

The meeting was called to order by Miss Hodgins who was unanimously elected Chairman pro-tem, Miss Kay Sheehan, Secretary pro-tem.

Miss Hodgins stated the call for the meeting and Mrs. Fife moved, seconded by Miss Aida Allwein, "That a National Association of Nurse Anesthetists be formed." Motion carried.

The Assembly also decided to affiliate with the American Nurses' Association.

Mrs. Fife, Miss Verna Rice and Miss Aida Allwein were appointed to draft a tentative copy of the Constitution and By-Laws. This report with . . . amendments was adopted:. . .

The committee on Constitution and By-Laws was instructed to see an attorney regarding the necessary procedure in acquiring a charter.

The charter members enrolled at the close of the meeting.

It was moved and seconded, "That the charter roll be left open until a later meeting that prospective members who were unavoidably detained may become charter members." Motion carried.

The election of permanent officers resulted as follows: President, Agatha C. Hodgins, nominated by Mrs. Fife. First Vice President . . . [Laura Davis], nominated by Miss Hodgins. Second Vice President, Miss Aida Allwein, nominated by Miss Kaiser. Third Vice President, Miss Helen Lamb, nominated by Miss Rice. Secretary, Mrs. . . . [Matilda Miller Root], nominated by Miss McFadden. Treasurer, Miss Verna Rice, nominated by Miss Allwein.

There being no further business the meeting adjourned at 5:30 P.M.[10] (emphasis added)

Given her intellectual conviction that nurse anesthesia service did not belong with nursing service, but rather should be a separate hospital service, why did Hodgins seek affiliation (comparable to that of the Red Cross, Public Health, and the National League of Nursing Education) with the American Nurses' Association? Her colleague Gertrude Fife years later suggested that "Hodgins realized they [the ANA] wouldn't allow that, but . . . she realized that the attempt should be made." Fife added that these developments "took years": "I went to Lakeside [in] 1924–1925, and I can remember Miss Hodgins talking about it very shortly after I arrived. Yet the meeting was not held until 1931. All that time it was a question of thinking and building."[11]

Considering the anger and resentment Hodgins still felt in 1941, it seems more likely that she did not see this rejection as inevitable, but had hoped to win the gratitude and affection of all nursing for delivering the "good news," the kerygma, of new horizons for the entire profession. A person with a less visionary sense of mission—and, perhaps, less ego—might have reacted the way another colleague, Miriam Shupp, did. For her, there was simply no reason to expect the nursing profession at large to be "ready to hear this. They weren't ready to accept the fact that nurses were doing this. . . . It just wasn't their field, and I couldn't see why she would think they would stand up and clap."[12] (It is interesting that the minutes of the first meeting read that the nurse anesthetists "decided to affiliate with the American Nurses' Association," not that they decided "to seek" affiliation.)

In any case, in November 1931 Hodgins began a rather lengthy correspondence, spanning a brief period of time, with the American Nurses' Association. The letters are revelatory of Hodgins's temperament. To its secretary she wrote (in a letter she later explained, that was "outlined by a Parliamentarian as we were most anxious to approach the matter in what was considered the proper way"):[13]

> The International Association of Nurse Anesthetists, recently organized with headquarters in Cleveland, Ohio, desires the privilege of affiliating with the American Nurses' Association. Therefore, the Association herewith makes formal application.[14]

Hodgins enclosed a copy of the Constitution, By-Laws, and Standing Rules, expressing the hope that the forthcoming ANA Biennial Convention in April 1932—less than six months away—would be the occasion of the affiliation. Hodgins's projected schedule, by its very brevity, suggests considerable optimism on her part.

A letter of reply from Marie Louis, chairman of the ANA's Revision and Membership Committee, in December 1931 expressed the need for further clarification on matters. For example, "I am not quite sure if I fully understand what you want. You speak of your organization as being international, and you ask affiliation with the American Nurses' Association, which is an organization composed of registered nurses residing in the United States or in possessions thereof."[15]

After receiving Louis's questions, Hodgins had the Constitution and Bylaws revised by an attorney. She sent Louis the revised material the following February. After noting that the new Association's name had, in fact, been changed to "*National* Association of Nurse Anesthetists," Hodgins set aside concern for parliamentarian protocol, and stated her purpose:

> The writer is well aware of existing conditions in regard to the number of nurse anesthetists in this country and also in other places. It is because of the increasing number of nurses interested in this particular work and growing realization of difficulties existing because of insufficient knowledge of, and proper emphasis on, the importance of education, that we who are most interested are

taking the steps to insure our ability to define and help maintain the status of the educated nurse anesthetist. This necessarily brings with it the effort to go on record as to educational standards necessary, before any nurse is legally entitled to administer anesthetic drugs. It also implies responsibility to work for such measures as will insure protection to properly qualified nurse anesthetists now engaged in this service.

You are doubtless aware that nurses with little or no education on the subject practicing anesthesia, is a serious cause of complex and disturbing difficulties constantly arising. This situation can only be cleared up by our ability to create a classification insuring protection to all concerned. Thus, briefly outlined, are the reasons leading to the organization.

Our reason for asking affiliation with the American Nurses' Association, is simply recognition of the primary fact that we are registered, graduate nurses, qualified for and pursuing a special work. This work being now our profession, we wish to emphasize it as our special concern, but also by affiliation with the American Nurses' Association to express in a public way our loyalty and interest in the larger group. This special service cannot be defined as nursing, but impinges closely upon and is irrevocably attached to the care of the sick.

In regard to the question of being a section, as the work is not nursing, we were of the opinion that section affiliation (if that is the proper term) would not be possible, but we are hopeful that recognition by and affiliation with the American Nurses' Association is a possible thing.[16]

On March 22, 1932, Hodgins, having not received a response to her letter sent five weeks earlier, wrote again not only to Louis ("We have had no reply and are, therefore, in doubt as to whether it reached you safely"),[17] but also once again to the ANA's assistant director, Alma Scott, summarizing the sequence of correspondence with the ANA since the previous November. Her letter contains the impatience and passion of a visionary:

To those who are interested and willing to work toward the establishment of future safeguarding of this important work and those engaged in it, encouragement and help from the American Nurses' Association will be of immeasurable value and in the final analysis, we can see nothing but mutual benefit to all as the result of such affiliation and help.[18]

The explanation from Scott, was written two days later:

I wish to acknowledge receipt of your letter of March 22, a copy of which has been sent to Miss Jane Van DeVrede, 131 Forrest Avenue, N.E., Atlanta, Georgia.

Miss Van DeVrede is now Chairman of the A.N.A. Revisions and Membership Committee. This appointment followed the resignation of Miss Marie Louis which was presented to the A.N.A. Board of Directors at the meeting held in January.

No doubt the letter which you wrote to Miss Louis, together with the revised copy of your Constitution and By-Laws, has been forwarded by Miss Louis to Miss Van DeVrede.

We know Miss Van DeVrede will be glad to get in touch with you as soon as she has information to send on to you.[19]

For Hodgins, the speed, courtesy, and reasonableness of the response did not signify. What she focused on was the fact that no indication was made of the imminent ANA convention, which *Hodgins* had targeted for the affiliation. She replied to Scott on March 28:

As no mention has been made of the nurse anesthetist group in the coming biennial convention at San Antonio, we presume that for this year the matter is in a tentative state. This, of course, is a disappointment to the many nurse anesthetists who have written to me in regard to this matter.[20]

The new Chairman, Van DeVrede, wrote to Hodgins on April 5. Hodgins's perception was correct: the nurse anesthetist affiliation was not on the convention agenda.

As you know, I have recently inherited the Committee on Revisions of the American Nurses' Association.

Your communications have been sent to the members of the Committee and should have been returned to me with recommendations before this, but the Committee members are separated by the length and breadth of the United States and it takes time.

Will you by chance be at the Biennial? If so, please get in touch with me at the Gunter Hotel.

This does not seem as simple a problem as on the surface it would appear, and it would be a help to talk things over, I am sure.[21]

Once again, Hodgins did not focus on any conciliatory features of the communication, but reacted to the failure of the ANA to meet *her* schedule for action. And, as she had made clear in her March 22 letter to Scott, she felt that the questions raised by the ANA had already been answered "satisfactorily." On April 7, she replied to Van De-

Vrede that she had canceled her plans to attend the convention and had reconsidered the affiliation:

> Your letter of April 5 received and the evident difficulties of putting the matter before a widely scattered committee are quite understood and appreciated.
>
> I deeply regret that no decision having been made by the American Nurses' Association in regard to the consideration of our problem, my original plan for attending the convention was changed. It is also evident from perusal of the Biennial Convention program that the pressing programs of nursing will fully occupy the time of those convening and, therefore, no real advantage will result from my attending.
>
> I am, however, arranging with some of the nurse anesthetists who I think may attend the convention, to get in touch with you at the Gunter Hotel and am hopeful that you will be able to go over the matter in a way that will be helpful to both groups.
>
> On analysis it would seem that our organization, being in a purely formative stage, the interests of the Association will be better served if no premature decisions are now made. We have incorporated the Association in the State of Ohio and feel hopeful of building up, within the next five years, an organization which will mean a great deal to the nurse anesthetist group and be a contributing factor toward enhancing the value and safety of anesthesia.[22]

As Hodgins wrote the following day to colleague Helen Lamb (whom she thought might attend the ANA meeting):

> As I have already stated to Miss [Verna] Rice, a small organization with high standards will accomplish our objectives more successfully than a larger one *half-heartedly* concerned with anesthesia and nursing.[23] (emphasis added)

Van DeVrede was not contacted by any nurse anesthetists during the convention. At its Board of Directors' meeting on April 9, the request for affiliation was rejected. The Board's position was that membership to the ANA was already available to nurse anesthetists "through their Alumnae, District and State Associations," and that these established avenues should continue to be utilized.[24]

The entire matter of a nurse anesthetist affiliation with the American Nurses' Association was raised and settled in *less than six months*. The results, however, were far-reaching. According to Ira Gunn:

> We in nursing have had our own civil war. Back in the late twenties and thirties, when the American Nurses' Association decided we

could not have our separate section within the association, the nurse anesthetists decided to form their own professional organization. Since that time we have been segregated. In most instances in civilian hospitals, the nurse anesthetist is responsible to the hospital administrator rather than to the nursing service administrator. And because we stopped communicating, the breach widened.[25]

Hodgins defended her position in a speech in June 1932 shortly after the ANA episode.[26] To a group of fellow anesthetists she said of "this immediate problem" regarding a "separate organization" for nurse anesthetists:

It means a clear acceptance of the fact that while anesthesia, by its very nature, impinges closely on surgery and less closely on nursing, . . . [it] is entitled to a place as a separate division of hospital service, its study being considered a distinct art and science.

She also lamented that "there is at present no place for our group, as such," adding that "we must therefore create this place and sooner done, the better." Yet, she admitted "that the present situation in regard to the 'status' of the nurse anesthetist is a confused and perplexing one, no intelligent person can deny."

Ironically, in this speech, Hodgins suggested an alternative source of support for the young organization, but, apparently, failed to grasp the significance of her own words:

It seems to us that anesthesia, being in no sense nursing, could not be absorbed into a strictly nursing group such as the A.N.A., as we hope to include in our sustaining membership surgeons, hospital superintendents, and others interested in advancing the cause.

It would, in fact, be an alliance with the American Hospital Association that would foster the profession of nurse anesthesia.

Agatha Hodgins suffered a heart attack on January 1, 1933. Whether because of her deteriorating health, or because of her inability to find a solution to the "perplexing" problem of professional organization, the new association was in a weak state: "When Miss Hodgins became ill, neither the first vice-president, Laura Davis, nor the secretary, Matilda Miller Root, was active. Verna Rice, the treasurer, was in Alabama, and the books were kept by Miriam Shupp at the University Hospitals in Cleveland. Except in name the Board of Management did not exist. The constitution and the bylaws were still far from being in a form that would be adaptable to the association's needs. No plans had been made for the first annual meeting. The total amount in the treasury was $492.25. . . . Less than 10 state affiliates were organized or in the process of organization."[27] As her successor Gertrude Fife later summed it up: "As far as the Association was concerned, everything was at a standstill."[28]

Fife also made clear in this memoir that it was John R. Mannix, then Assistant Director of University Hospitals, who played the crucial role: "John Mannix was an organizer. He was interested in the development of the hospital, and, incidentally, he was the one that started the Blue Cross plan. . . . John Mannix is largely responsible for our organization. . . . He was a driver, he was king pin, he was boss." He was also the Administrator in charge of the Anesthesia Department. In the wake of Hodgins's illness, Fife had been appointed temporary head: "In one of my first conferences with Mr. Mannix he told me that the one thing he insisted that I do was to get the Association going." Fife protested that she "didn't know anything about organization. He said, 'I'll help you,' and he helped us with the first meeting." At the time, Fife had no position in the sequence of authority in the Association. Mannix helped her circumvent that obstacle: "He told me to call a meeting of the Cleveland anesthetists and have them vote me secretary, or whatever you would call it, to get the first meeting started."

In early May 1933 Mannix then wrote to Bert W. Caldwell, MD, executive secretary of the American Hospital Association. The letter voiced his appreciation of the significance of nurse anesthetists to the nation's health-care system:

> Mrs. Gertrude Fife, who is assistant director of our School of Anesthesia and who is also secretary of the National Association of Nurse Anesthetists, has spoken to me regarding the possibility of the Anesthesia Association holding their meeting in Milwaukee simultaneously with the meeting of the American Hospital Association and I suggested that she communicate with you.
>
> The Association which Mrs. Fife represents is a new organization, only about two years of age, but which has already a paid membership of three hundred and sixty-two. The association has members from coast to coast. Inasmuch as this group plays a very important part in the present day hospitalization, I believe it would be well if arrangements could be made whereby their meetings could regularly be held while the American Hospital Association meetings are in session.[29]

There was ample precedent for Mannix's suggestion. For example, the May 1933 issue of the *Bulletin of the American Hospital Association* noted that four other health-care associations were already scheduled to meet in September along with the American Hospital Association:

the American Protestant Hospital Association, the American Occupational Therapy Association, the American Association of Hospital Social Workers, and the Children's Hospital Association of America.

Caldwell's speedy response showed that the National Association of Nurse Anesthetists would be a welcomed addition. To Fife, he wrote on May 10:

> The American Hospital Association would particularly welcome an arrangement of this kind and believes that it would have many mutual benefits which members of your Association and ours could enjoy.[30]

Caldwell's next paragraph underlined the fact that he shared Mannix's perception of the importance, the essential contribution, of nurse anesthetists to the hospital system:

> You are, of course, aware that a very large percentage of the hospitals are employing nurse anesthetists—this in spite of the very insistent movement to confine the administration of anesthetics or at least to have the department of anesthesia in every hospital under the control of a doctor of medicine. We are in no means in sympathy with this last mentioned movement, and I am sure that the hospitals would come to a very much better understanding as to the problems of nurse anesthetists if the two meetings could be held concurrently in the same city. . . . I will be particularly glad to go into this matter further with you and I assure you that we will make every arrangement possible for a very successful meeting for your Association.[31]

The practice of concurrent meetings of health-care groups was common—ironically, for example, the 1932 biennial meeting of the American Nurses' Association in San Antonio that Hodgins had hoped would approve affiliation with her National Association of Nurse Anesthetists was not only held with the National League of Nursing Education, but was scheduled concurrently with the Texas Hospital Association meeting. In view of Hodgins's insistence on nurse anesthesia being considered a separate "hospital service" rather than part of "nursing," it is, again, strange that she did not consider an alliance with the hospital group.

Mannix played another pivotal role in the development of the National Association of Nurse Anesthetists. As mentioned above, the organization had been ineffectively constructed. As Miriam Shupp described it, "They had some kind of unwieldy board. . . . I don't know how many people were on it. . . . Probably everybody that belonged to the Association was on the Board."[32] But, once again, on the advice of Mannix "the constitution and the bylaws of the American Hospital Association and of the Ohio Hospital Association were used as models for revising the association's organizational structure in order that power could be concentrated in a small board of trustees."[33]

Planning the convention program was another task that fell to Fife: "We were going to put on the first convention. Who was going to make out the program? We had very little time. And Mannix said that we had to meet . . . we had to put that convention on. And, consequently, Helen [Lamb] and Walter [Powell] came to Cleveland and we made out the program over my kitchen . . . my dining room table. The three of us."[34]

Like all the work that Fife took up (and her contribution would be herculean), she—along with the brilliant Lamb and the éminence grise, Walter Powell—produced a success. The program was printed in the September 1933 issue of *The Bulletin of the American Hospital Association:*

First Annual Meeting
of the
National Association of Nurse Anesthetists

For several years there has been a growing conviction in the minds of the nurse anesthetists that organization into a coherent group pledged to carry out certain objectives would result in the progress of the work. As a result, on June 17, 1931, an organization meeting was held at Lakeside Hospital, Cleveland, Ohio.

The meeting was attended by forty-nine nurse anesthetists, representing twelve states. The total number interested in the formation of such an organization, but who were unable to attend the meeting, was 125, representing forty-two states.

Since this time the work of organization has been steadily going forward, and at the present writing our membership has increased to 452.

We feel that we have been most fortunate in the arrangement, whereby we can meet concurrently with the American Hospital Association. This connection will help us to achieve our objectives, as follows:

(1) To advance the science and art of anesthesiology.
(2) To develop educational standards and technique in the administration of anesthetic drugs.
(3) To facilitate efficient coöperation between nurse anesthetists and

the medical profession, hospitals, and other agencies interested in anesthesiology.

(4) To establish and maintain a central bureau for information, reference, and assistance in matters pertaining to the science and art of anesthesiology.

(5) To promulgate an educational program to enlighten the general public as to the importance of the proper administration of anesthetics, and to take all proper steps to accomplish, as nearly as possible, complete protection to the public, as well as to protect the professional rights of the Association and its members.

PROGRAM
Milwaukee, Wisconsin
September 13–15, 1933

Wednesday, September 13
8:00 A.M. Registration—Auditorium
9:00 A.M. Clinic—St. Joseph's Hospitals, 5000 W. Chambers St.
　　　　 Address by Dr. Chester Echols
　　　　　　 St. Joseph's Hospital
　　　　　　 (following Clinic at St. Joseph's Hospital)
12:30 P.M. Luncheon—Hotel Astor
　　　　 Letter of Greeting—
　　　　　　 Dr. Evarts Graham
　　　　　　　　 Professor of Surgery
　　　　　　　　 Washington University

2:00 P.M. General Session:
　　　　 (1) President's Address—
　　　　　　 Agatha C. Hodgins
　　　　　　　　 Director Post-Graduate School of Anesthesia
　　　　　　　　 University Hospitals of Cleveland
　　　　 (2) The Importance of a Well Organized Anesthesia
　　　　 Department
　　　　　　 Malcolm T. MacEachern, M.D., C.M.
　　　　　　　　 Director of Hospital Activities
　　　　　　　　 American College of Surgeons
　　　　 (3) The Value of the Nurse Anesthetist to Present-Day
　　　　 Hospitalization
　　　　　　 Bert W. Caldwell, M.D.
　　　　　　　　 Executive Secretary
　　　　　　　　 American Hospital Association
　　　　 (4) The Future of the Nurse Anesthetist
　　　　　　 Gertrude L. Fife

University Hospitals of Cleveland
Discussion

Wednesday Evening   Banquet and Ball
Wisconsin Club Gardens

Thursday, September 14
9:00 A.M. Tour of the City
12:30 P.M. Luncheon at Hotel Wisconsin
2:00 P.M. General Session:
  (1) (Topic to be announced)
      Mr. Robert Jolly
      Superintendent Memorial Hospital, Houston, Tex.
  (2) The Induction of an Anesthetic
      Ruth M. Nash
      Director, Post Graduate School of Anesthesia
      Long Island College Hospital
      Brooklyn, N.Y.
  (3) Intratracheal Anesthesia
      Helen Lamb
      Director, Post Graduate School of Anesthesia
      Barnes Hospital, St. Louis, Mo.
  Discussion
4:00 P.M. Business Session—(Active and Associate members of the
      National Association of Nurse Anesthetists)
6:30 P.M. Dinner—Plankinton Hotel
      After-dinner Conference
  (1) Ethylene Anesthesia
      Catherine Cameron
      Director, Post Graduate School of Anesthesia
      St. Joseph's Hospital, Milwaukee, Wis.
  (2) Carbon Dioxide Filtration Anesthesia
      Rosalie McDonald,
      Chief Anesthetist
      Emory University Hospital
      Atlanta, Georgia
  Discussion

Friday, September 15
8:00 A.M. Breakfast meeting of Officers and Board of Trustees—
      Plankinton Hotel

By the close of the convention, even the modest Fife (newly elected second President of the Association) would declare, "I feel that we are making history, and that we are laying the foundation for a fine organization, that will be of great benefit to the future of the work."[35]

A letter of welcome from Dr. Evarts Graham, Professor of Surgery, Washington University, St. Louis (for whom Lamb acted as anesthetist), was read to the members. It voiced the continued support of nurse anesthetists by surgeons of prominence:

Miss Helen Lamb has told me of this first meeting of your Association and has asked me to write a letter of greeting. I feel that I am highly honored in being asked to do so. One of the most important contributions towards the perfection of surgery has been the improvement in the conduction of anesthesia. *To a large extent I feel that the skillful, well-trained nurse anesthetist has been responsible for the great improvement in the practice of anesthesia which one sees throughout this country now as compared with twenty years ago.* In order to continue the excellent work which has already been started, it is wise to have an organization such as has been created in order to establish certain minimum standards of training and efficiency. No stigma can be attached to the nurse anesthetist if she proves worthy of her position. It will be necessary for your leaders to safeguard your profession by recognizing the able and not recognizing the improperly trained anesthetist.

There is need for an organization such as you have founded. I hope that it will have a long life and a prosperous one.[36] (emphasis added)

"The Value of the Nurse Anesthetist to Present-Day Hospitalization" was the topic of Dr. Bert W. Caldwell, Executive Secretary of the American Hospital Association. As noted above, he had already communicated to Fife his support of nurse anesthetists, even in the face of pressure from the physician-anesthetist-led anti–nurse movement. In this paper he gave a pragmatic assessment of the situation: "There will always be a wide field of endeavor, and at fair remuneration, for the nurse anesthetist. Many of our best surgeons are employing their services in our best hospitals. It is unlikely that there will ever be a sufficiently large number of medical anesthetists to fill the requirements of the hospitals which are now employing nurse anesthetists, or meet the wishes of the surgeons who prefer the services of the nurse anesthetist."[37] Not surprisingly, hospital administrator Caldwell addressed the subject of the structure of the hospital anesthesia department, in effect sharing Hodgins's view that anesthetists did not fall under "nursing service":

The department of anesthesia in every hospital should be under the direction of a skilled and experienced anesthetist, directly responsible to the surgical division. The anesthetist is the assistant and the cooperator with the surgeon in all of his work necessitating the administration of an anesthetic.[38]

Caldwell's comments also make clear that, in 1933, anesthesia was still viewed as the "handmaid" of surgery.

Hodgins, unable to be present because of her illness, nevertheless provided a "President's Address." There is a touching self-consciousness about her language, probably a result of her desire to provide lofty, significant words for the occasion which she, more than anyone else, realized to be a momentous one:

It is a matter for felicitation that the American Hospital Association courteously extended to our new Association an invitation to meet with them—a privilege happily accepted and much appreciated. Your president greatly regrets that at this significant gathering, her greetings and good wishes for a successful and profitable meeting must, perforce, be delegated to another. This present meeting is the first-fruit of what might be called an adventure. That adventuring is a necessary and vital thing to life and growth is a sound principle, emphasized by our wisest philosophers, "There never can be any static maintenance of perfection—advance or decadence are the only choices offered to mankind." [Whitehead] This spirit of adventure is then the dynamic force that keeps us constantly contrasting what we are and what we may be and supplies the necessary courage to change from static to growing condition.[39]

In the concluding paragraph of her paper, Hodgins summarized the spiritual disposition she had urged her colleagues to embrace. She here effectively used the metaphor of her home in Cape Cod, where she wrote in forced retirement:

The house I now live in is well over the century mark. Built in far-off Colonial days, it has, while lending itself to changes necessary for our more modern ideas of comfort, retained the original characteristics of beauty, simplicity and usefulness. Let us keep our abiding faith, that each component group, now building their part of our organization, may so embody in their work the spiritual qualities of courage, simplicity, endurance and good judgement that the integral whole may, like this little house, give warmth, light and security to the present generation and be of continuing beauty and usefulness to generations coming after us.[40]

It was left to Fife, whom fate had cast in the critical leadership position of the young, national organization, to address the most pressing, practical issue facing nurse anesthetists: "We must . . . make an earnest effort to standardize the education of the nurse anesthetist."[41] Fife, with the benefit of some expert *physician* advice, outlined the necessary course of action, one in which nurse anesthetists would take control over their own accelerating professionalization:

> The first step in the program was made when we organized in June of 1931. Our second step in the program is to give assurance that our members are and will be only those who by reason of their training, experience, knowledge and character are qualified to undertake the work before us.

She then called for a committee to investigate all schools of nurse anesthesia with the object of creating a list of "accredited" schools because the National Association "should at all times be able to furnish information to hospitals or surgeons desirous of employing anesthetists regarding the standing of schools and the qualifications of members of the National Association desirous of obtaining positions."

Finally, there would be "the establishment of national board examinations for nurse anesthetists" that "would place in the surgeon's hands an official record showing that her knowledge of the subject has met with the approval of an examining board—a board chosen and functioning to safeguard the surgeon's interest, the interest of the hospitals, and the interest of the public."[42]

Thus, in 1933, the agenda was set. Unfortunately some factors beyond the control of the Association—including another world war—would delay its implementation. But, then, Hodgins had warned, nurse anesthetists would need "endurance."

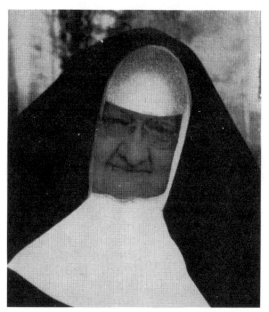

1. Sister Secundina Mindrup (1868–1951), an
early nurse anesthetist. The recruitment of
religious hospital sisters into anesthesia began in the late 1870s by surgeons who
needed anesthetists committed to patient
care without concern for financial reward or
career advancement. (AANA)

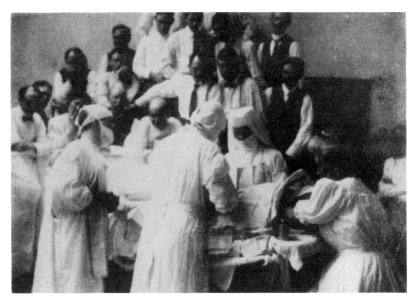

2. An early surgery at St. Mary's Hospital, Rochester, Minnesota, founded in
   1889. Drs. W. J. Mayo and C. H. Mayo are assisted by Sister Joseph and an
   unidentified anesthetist, probably Alice Magaw. (Mayo Clinic)

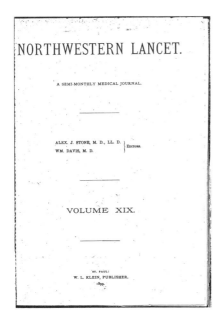

3. Magaw's first published paper,
   "Observations in Anesthesia," a
   report on over three thousand
   cases, appeared in the *Northwestern Lancet* in 1899. (John
   Crerar Library)

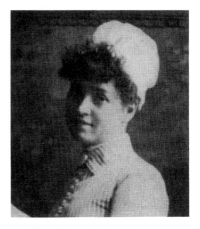

4. Alice Magaw (AANA)

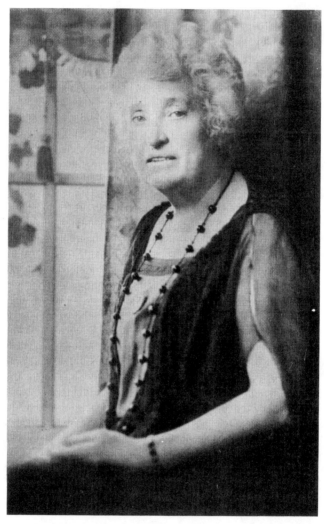

5. Alice Magaw Kessel (1860–1928), anesthetist to Drs. William J. and Charles H. Mayo, who referred to her as "the Mother of Anesthesia." (AANA)

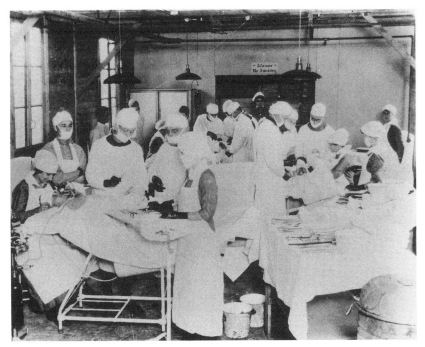

6. Nurse anesthetists serve in Base Hospital No. 52, Haute Marne, France, 1918. (US Army Center of Military History)

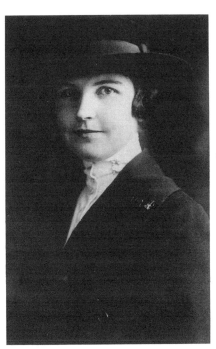

7. Sophie Gran Winton (1887– 1989) was awarded the *Croix de Guerre* for her service as a nurse anesthetist in Mobile Hospital No. 1 in the Chateau-Thierry area of France. (AANA)

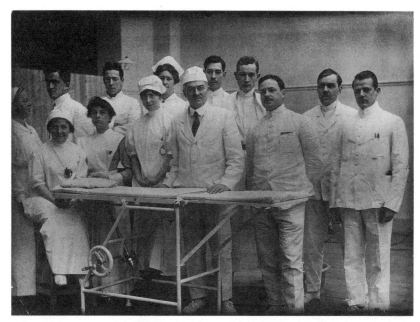

8. Dr. George W. Crile with his Lakeside Unit, American Ambulance, January 13, 1915. Agatha Hodgins is seated at the left. (AANA)

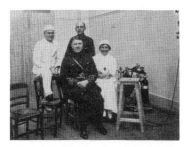

9. Dr. Crile, British surgeon Sir Berkeley Moynihan (seated), Captain Leonard Braithwaite, and Agatha Hodgins. (AANA)

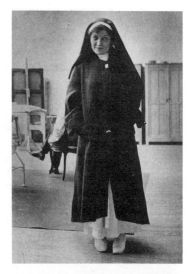

10. Agatha Cobourg Hodgins (1877–1945), founder of the National Association of Nurse Anesthetists (in 1939 changed to the American Association of Nurse Anesthetists). (AANA)

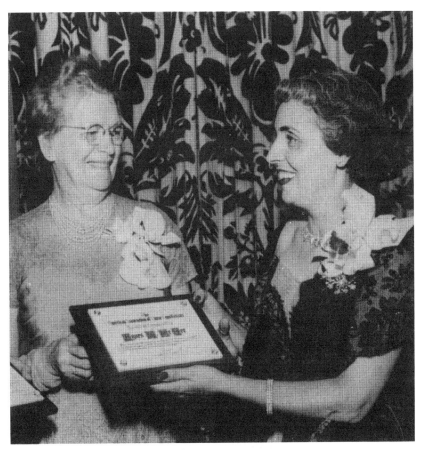

11. Agnes McGee receives the AANA Award of Appreciation from President Josephine (Bonnie) Bunch in 1953 for organizing the first postgraduate course in nurse anesthesia at St. Vincent's Hospital, Portland, Oregon, in 1909. (AANA)

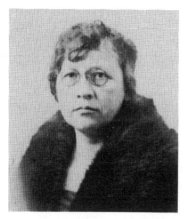

12. Anna Marie S. Rose (AANA)

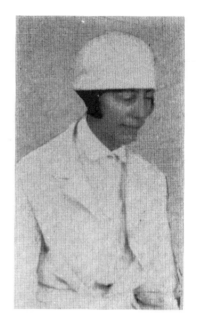

13. Margaret Boise (AANA)

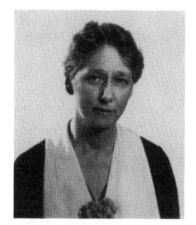

14. Alice M. Hunt (AANA)

In the first two decades of the twentieth century, the achievements of individual nurse anesthetists contributed to acceptance of the nursing specialty. For example, in 1909 Marie Rose was appointed anesthetist to the General Surgical Clinic of the University of Pennsylvania Hospital, where she also taught anesthesia to both medical students and other nurses. Margaret Boise, in collaboration with surgeon Hugh H. Young, invented a gas-ether machine later known as the Boise–Young apparatus. Head anesthetist for the surgical department of the Johns Hopkins Hospital, she also came to administer anesthetics for most of the patients of William Stewart Halsted. Alice Hunt, in 1922, was appointed instructor in anesthesia with university rank at the Yale Medical School, where she taught nurses and medical students for twenty-six years. (AANA)

NATIONAL ASSOCIATION OF NURSE ANESTHETISTS

CHARTER MEMBERS

June 17, 1931

15

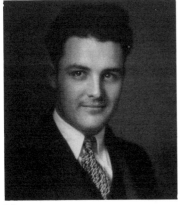

16

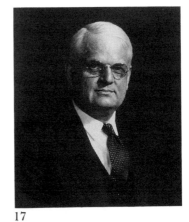

17

Essential support for the young National Association of Nurse Anesthetists came from administrators and physicians of University Hospitals of Cleveland such as John Robert Mannix (left) and Carl Henri Lenhart, MD. (University Hospitals of Cleveland)

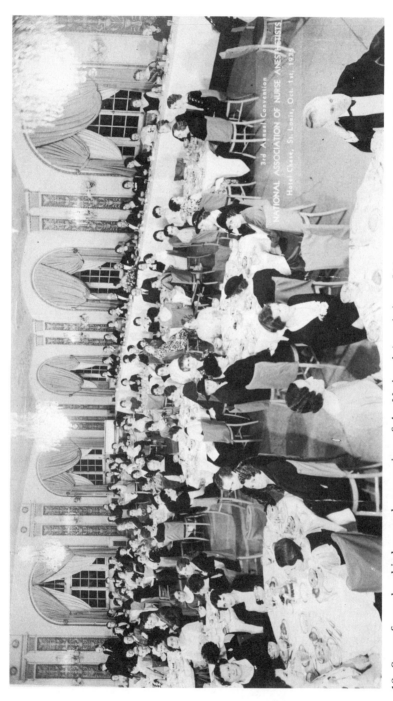

18. Scene from the third annual convention of the National Association of Nurse Anesthetists, held in St. Louis on October 1, 1935. (AANA)

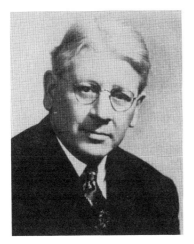

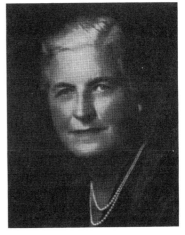

19. Verne C. Hunt, MD (AANA)   20. Dagmar Nelson (AANA)

The legality of nurse anesthetists was definitively established through the 1934 trial of Dagmar Nelson. The support of surgeons such as Dr. Hunt played a crucial role in the victory.

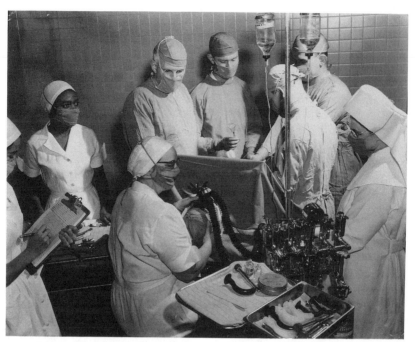

21. Dr. Evarts A. Graham, a father of modern chest surgery, with his nurse anesthetist, Helen Lamb. She served two terms as AANA president, 1940–42. (AANA)

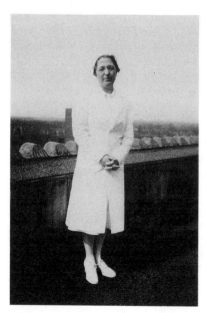

22. Gertrude LaBrake Fife, nurse anesthetist for pioneering heart surgeon Claude S. Beck. When Agatha Hodgins became ill, Fife assumed the burden of developing the young National Association of Nurse Anesthetists. (AANA)

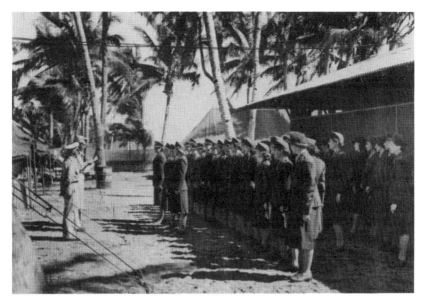

23. Nurse anesthetist Annie Mealer, AANA member, is among this group of Army nurses shown after their release from a three-year imprisonment by the Japanese in the Philippines. (US Army Signal Corps)

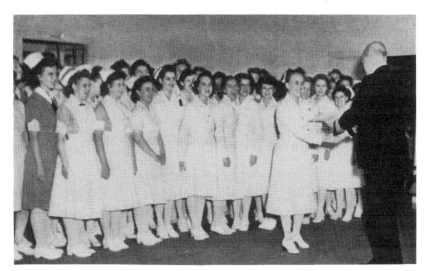

24. Lieutenant (j.g.) Ruth Toenberg, NC, USNR, AANA member, receives a citation for meritorious service on board a US hospital ship sailing in enemy waters from November 1943 to April 1945. (AANA)

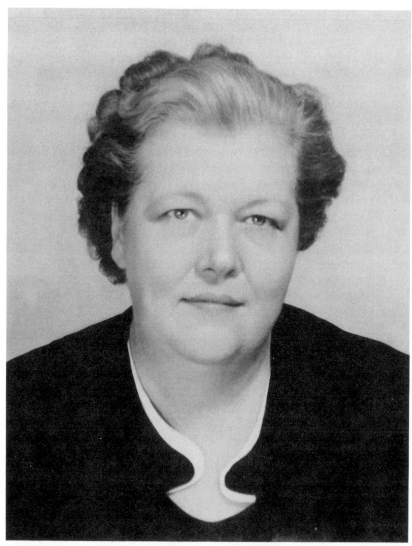

25. Florence A. McQuillen, CRNA, Executive Director of the American Association of Nurse Anesthetists, 1948–70. No single Association leader before or after "Mac" would exercise comparable control over all facets of its business. (AANA)

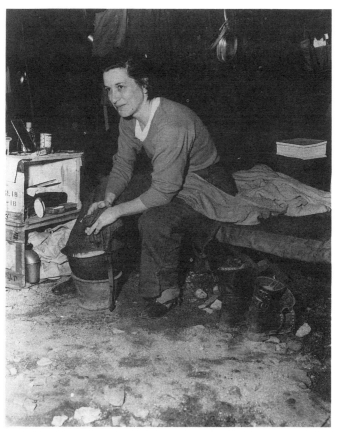

26. Captain Jane Thurness, AANA member, serving with the first MASH Unit in Korea, 1950–51. (Jane Thurness)

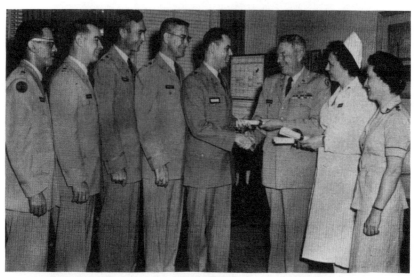

27. The first all-male class to complete the year-long course in anesthesiology for nurses at Walter Reed General Hospital, Washington, DC, receives diplomas in 1961 from Brigadier General Floyd L. Wergeland, hospital commander. Lieutenant Colonel Ruth P. Satterfield, CRNA, course director, and Lieutenant Colonel Elizabeth Jane Thurness, CRNA, assistant director, congratulate the "Ethernauts." (US Army)

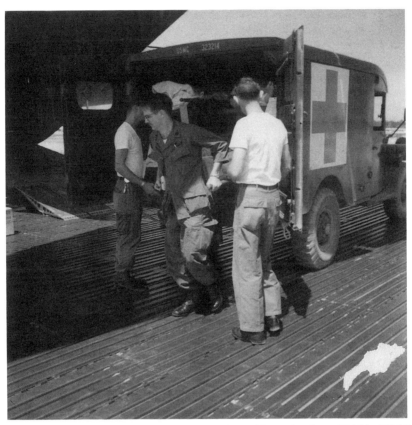

28. Nurse anesthetist Lieutenant Colonel David R. Fletcher, CRNA, USAF, NC (center), works in the 903rd Aeromedical Evacuation Squadron transporting fresh battle casualties at Quang Tri, Vietnam, in 1968. (David R. Fletcher)

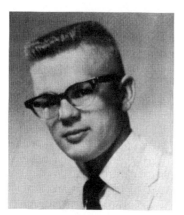

29. Lieutenant Jerome E.
    Olmsted, CRNA (AANA)

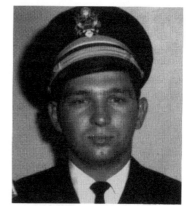

30. Lieutenant Kenneth R.
    Shoemaker, Jr., CRNA
    (AANA)

Of the ten nurses who lost their lives in the Vietnam conflict, two were nurse anesthetists. First lieutenants Olmsted and Shoemaker, assigned to the 67th Evacuation Hospital at Qui Nhon, were killed in the crash of a C-47 transport plane carrying wounded from Pleiku to Qui Nhon.

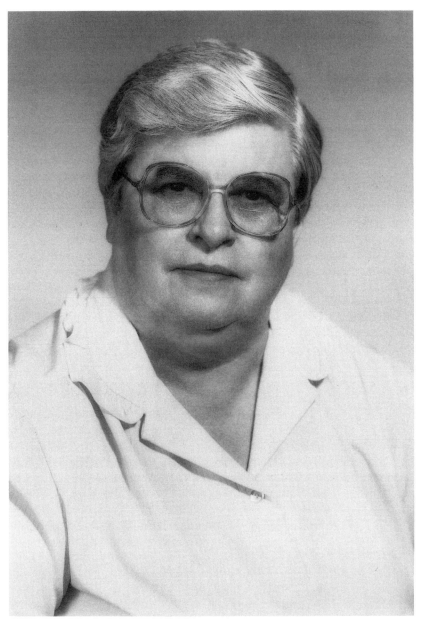

31. Ira P. Gunn, CRNA, MLN, FAAN (LTC, USA, retired), has distinguished herself in many areas relating to nurse anesthesia, including practice, research, education, publications, consultation, credentialing, and government relations. (AANA)

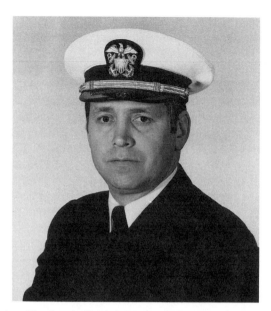

34. Commander Charles A. Reese, CRNA, NC, USN, Medical Department, *U.S.S. Nimitz.* Reese was decorated for his life-saving activities on the aircraft carrier when, on May 26, 1981, one of the ship's jets crashed onto its landing deck, killing 14 persons and injuring 48. (US Navy)

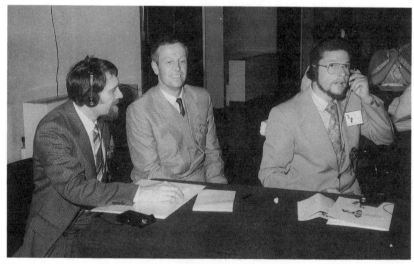

35. Fritz Knecht (left), President of the Swiss association of nurse anesthetists, Hermi Lohnert, and Gustave Mueller at the First International Symposium for Nurse Anesthetists held in Lucerne, Switzerland, in 1985. (Ronald F. Caulk)

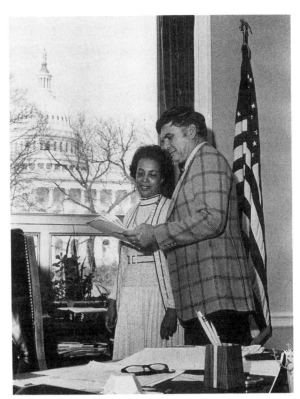

32. AANA President 1973–74, Goldie D. Brangman, CRNA, first black president of the Association, in the Washington office of US Representative Al Ulmann (D. Ore), vice-chairman of the House Ways and Means Committee. AANA membership of black women was approved in 1944. (AANA)

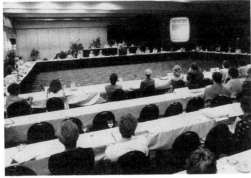

33. A meeting of the National Federation for Specialty Nursing Organizations, founded in 1973. The AANA is a charter member. (AANA)

· 5 ·

Worlds at War

You people have been rather on the spot for the past three or four years because you have been taking away, so it is said, from starving physicians what may be transferred into a valuable consultation service. Now that offices are filling and practice is picking up, I think probably the crisis of the situation has passed.
—J. C. Doane, MD (1937)[1]

A s Medical Director of Jewish Hospital, Philadelphia, Dr. Doane was familiar with the recent crises faced by nurse anesthetists. It was at this hospital that Hilda Salomon, noted above, was practicing with great distinction while she also held office in the National Association of Nurse Anesthetists, as First Vice-President in 1934, and as President in 1935 and 1936. She was, in 1937, in the first of her three years as an Association Trustee.

Doane's description of nurse anesthetists being "rather on the spot" was an effort at humorous understatement. Fueled by the economic pressures of the great Depression, anti-nurse anesthetist activities had been intensified, culminating in 1934 in the test case of Dagmar Nelson. The outcome of her trial in California—to a considerable degree affected by the supportive "expert witness" of surgeons—definitively established the legality of nurse anesthetists. Meanwhile, in Cleveland, the young National Association of Nurse Anesthetists continued with what had been *its* priority from the beginning: the development and implementation of its education programs. These plans (already hampered because of scarce financial resources) were further disrupted by World War II. It not only brought a call to military and a greatly increased civilian service, but also brought the considerable complication of the wartime emergency-trained anesthetist.

Medicine's Internecine Conflict

From the earliest discussions of the need for a professional anesthetist in the nineteenth century, medical economics was an explicit issue:

the inability of physicians to earn a living in anesthesia, the difficulty in collecting anesthesia fees (often involving a criticism of the surgeon in this matter), the professional dead-end anesthesia represented for the medical graduate. And from the earliest days of physician-organized anti-nurse anesthetist activity in the twentieth century, objection to their existence was formulated as a violation of medical "property rights" and an "economic crime" against physicians. Paul Starr has written of the conflict, full-blown by the 1930s, "within medicine itself, the division of labor between specialists and general practitioners. . . . When specialists claimed that various techniques and procedures required their skills, general practitioners often found themselves damned in the same breath as nonphysicians."[2] The difference in the field of anesthesia, however, was that the growing body of physician-specialists needed and wanted the general practitioner in the field (if only as an occasional anesthetist) in order to gather the numerical strength necessary to claim the field for medicine. Anesthetics, by the 1930s, had reached significant economic proportions. Reflecting on this fact in 1938, Dr. Henry Hedden observed:

> Someone recently stated that there were probably 5,000,000 paid-for anesthesias administered every year in the United States by nurse anesthetists. I estimate that this represents a potential cash income of $50,000,000.00 to $75,000,000.00, so is it any wonder that when the doctors realize this, they should hope to recapture the field of endeavor which they have spurned and scorned in a large measure as being unworthy of their professional attainments?[3]

In this war against nurse anesthetists, a unified physician front was never achieved. There were too many surgeons who favored, defended, and depended upon nurse anesthetists.

An early, and ironic, indication of disagreement between some surgeons and some physician-anesthetists appears in the August 1914 issue of the *American Journal of Surgery,* which contains—on the same page as its announcement of its forthcoming quarterly *Anesthesia Supplement,* to be edited by McMechan—an editorial titled, "Nurses as Anesthetists." It is a nonemotional description of the present state of practice regarding the use of nurse anesthetists. Noting that "In many large hospitals, private and public, the function of administering anesthetics has been delegated to a non-medical person," and that the "legal status of trained nurses, insofar as the administration of anesthetics is concerned, has not been defined by law," it addresses the argument "that a general medical training is essential to develop a careful and efficient anesthetist" with what it calls "the practical answer":

The practical answer is found in the experience of large hospitals wherein nurses have been very successfully employed as anesthetists. If practically their employment has been advantageous to the surgical service *without in the slightest degree endangering the patients*, it is difficult to maintain that nurses with a lack of medical training cannot be efficient anesthetists. (emphasis added)

For this editorial in the *American Journal of Surgery*, the matter of nurse anesthetists is one to be settled by the community of surgeons itself, with "little necessity for arguing with legislatures nor for blaming the community":

There is only one question involved: "Do surgeons desire nurses to administer anesthetics?" If the answer be in the affirmative, the laws should be altered so as to include the administration of anesthetics within the activities delegated to the nursing profession. If surgeons are opposed to nurses as anesthetists, no legislation is necessary. It merely remains with the profession to discontinue the use of nurses in this capacity and to discourage their employment in hospitals, private institutions and private practice.

The matter of "medical economics" and property rights did not go unaddressed in this column. Interestingly, its placing the welfare of the community above private interest would be echoed in the *Frank v. South* decision:

From the standpoint of medical economics, there is naturally objection to the preemption of any part of medical work by others than physicians. In the development of social progress, however, the welfare of the community alone is considered and the particular disadvantage to any particular profession receives but little consideration.[4]

But, as was discussed above, and it bears repeating in this context, McMechan would use the pages of the *Anesthesia Supplement* to the *American Journal of Surgery* to recommend strategies for the abolition of the "present menace of the nurse anesthetist," urging "that the Medical Practice Acts of the various States be so amended" as to achieve that end. Taking a stand opposed to the *American Journal of Surgery's* own, McMechan called it "imperative" that "medical associations should question the ethical standing of those surgeons who persist in employing lay-anesthetists [read "nurse anesthetists"], in the presence of competent, licensed practitioners [read "physicians"], who are ready to undertake the work and shoulder its full responsibilities."[5]

Two months later, the never-reticent McMechan again challenged the surgeons in his *Supplement* to their own *Journal*. In the July 1915 issue, mentioned earlier, he elaborated on the tension between pro-nurse anesthetist surgeons and anti-nurse anesthetist physicians in his editorial, "The American College of Surgeons and Unlicensed Anesthetists":

> The drastic attitude of the American College of Surgeons toward *fee-splitting* loses much of its force in view of the fact that the organization permits some of its most prominent members to continue the routine employment of unlicensed anesthetists. (original emphasis)

For McMechan, this policy was "in direct violation of the letter and spirit of all *Medical Practice Acts*." Therefore, he declared, "The nurse-anesthetist must go because she is unlicensed, and because her employment is as much an economic crime against the profession and public as *fee-splitting*," and that the American College of Surgeons, at its next meeting, "take action in this matter [of outlawing nurse anesthetists]," or "stand convicted of playing favorites, violating medical ethics and, alienating a certain proportion of licensed practitioners [read 'physicians'] from a legitimate source of financial support"[6] from the occasional administration of anesthetics.

How these pressures affected individual nurse anesthetists can be appreciated by examining the experiences of four such practitioners—all activities occurring in California, site of the Nelson trial. As has been noted, physician anesthetist societies increased during the 1920s. The Pacific Coast Association of Anesthetists was organized in 1922, and was given a Section on Anesthesia within the California Medical Society that same year.[7] It is not surprising, then, that Hodgins noted, in 1922, that in California

> [A] marked reaction against the nurse anesthetist was reported, and a good deal of pressure was being brought to bear in a great number of hospitals who were employing the nurse anesthetists. The strongest objection seemed to be against nurse anesthetists who were working on the fee basis; this being apparently most strongly objected to by the "specialists" in anesthesia.[8]

Sophie Gran Winton, discussed earlier in connection with her highly decorated World War I nurse anesthetist service, moved to California after the war because the climate was more healthful for her ailing husband. Welcomed by her mentor from Swedish Hospital in Minneapolis, G. W. Olson, then Assistant Superintendent of Los Angeles County General Hospital—who had persuaded her to enter the field—she nevertheless encountered the significant anti-nurse anesthetist activity in that area, and never practiced in a hospital. She became a partner in a private dental clinic, published research on dental anesthesia, and was honored by the Mexican Dental Society in association with the International Dental Association for her work in advancing the field of dental anesthesia. She later opened an out-patient plastic surgery clinic in Hollywood, attending some of the most notable film celebrities of the era. Winton's reaction to the anti–nurse anesthetist activity, so dramatically ironic in her case, was to become an independent practitioner. She would also play a significant part in supporting the rights of other nurse anesthetists to work in hospitals by helping form the first California Association of Nurse Anesthetists, serving as its first president, and by her moral and financial support of Dagmar Nelson in her trial.[9]

The situation in California intensified when, through the influence of the physician anesthetists, the California State Board of Medical Examiners adopted the following resolution in March 1928:

> *Whereas,* It has been called to the attention of the Board of Medical Examiners that a number of physicians and surgeons and hospitals throughout the State of California permit anaesthetics to be administered by persons not licensed to do so under the Medical Practice Act, such administration of anaesthetics by such unlicensed persons constituting violations of the Medical Practice Act, now, therefore,

> *Be It Resolved* That, inasmuch as the administration of anaesthetics by persons not licensed under the Medical Practice Act constitutes a violation of said Act, the Secretary of the Board of Medical Examiners be, and he is hereby, requested to give notice to physicians and surgeons and hospitals in order that physicians and surgeons and hospitals may govern themselves accordingly; and

> *Be It Further Resolved* That the publication of this resolution in *California and Western Medicine* shall constitute such notice to Physicians and Surgeons, and

> *Be It Further Resolved* That the mailing of this resolution to hospitals shall constitute notice to said hospitals.[10]

When the Highland Hospital of Alameda County received this communication—challenging the right of its nurse anesthetist, Eva Wilson, a graduate nurse of the Samuel Merritt Hospital School of Nursing, Oakland, California, to administer anesthetics—it moved to defend her. Noting the excellence of her work, Dr. Benjamin W. Black, director of the institution, said:

[She] is acknowledged by all the surgeons as probably the best anesthetist in this section. . . . Not only is she a good anesthetist herself and by preference would be the anesthetist for most of the surgeons who operate, but remarkable as it sounds, she has been able to teach internes to their satisfaction and at the conclusion of the interne year has given a definite course of instruction with demonstration in anesthesia so that the internes have left the hospital not only feeling a great deal of respect for her, but feeling that she is as skillful as any one could expect.[11]

Dr. Black therefore took the matter to the District Attorney and asked for a ruling on the legality of Wilson's practice. The result was a finding that "the anesthetist was under active orders while giving anesthetics, of the operating surgeon, and was not practicing medicine independently." Dr. Black even offered to be party to a "friendly" suit "if such were the desire" of the Attorney General. But nothing more came of the matter. Dr. Black concluded: "Dr. Harry Smith, who specializes in anesthesia, is the chief of the department of anesthesia but except for demonstration and teaching purposes he does not give anesthetics but is quite satisfied as are the surgeons here, with the work of Miss Wilson."[12]

Yet a different reaction came from a similar move against another nurse anesthetist. Adeline Curtis, a graduate of the Providence Hospital School of Nursing, Seattle, had been a staff anesthetist at the Johnston-Wickett Clinic, Anaheim, since 1921. Working in Orange County, she gave anesthetics for three surgeons in four different hospitals. When the clinic was notified in March 1928 of the resolution of the State Board of Medical Examiners, Curtis stopped her anesthesia work, performed office duties at the clinic, and launched her own legal investigation that spanned several months and cost her several thousand dollars. She hired her own attorney, Thomas L. McFadden, of Anaheim, to discover the reality of California law regarding the administration of anesthetics. Curtis was rehired as a clinic anesthetist in December, 1928, when McFadden stated that her anesthetic work was not in violation of California law.

Armed with this finding, Curtis began spreading the word to other nurse anesthetists in the Southern California area, visiting hospitals and giving lectures. She also began urging the nurse anesthetists to organize. In February 1930 the first meeting of the California Association of Nurse Anesthetists was held in Los Angeles. Thirteen members were present at the second meeting, held in Anaheim, and Sophie Gran Winton was elected president. Curtis, in touch with Agatha Hodgins regarding matters of state and national organization, was less than happy with Hodgins's request to delay any continued organization of state groups until the National Association of Nurse Anesthetists founded in Cleveland had finalized its bylaws. Curtis felt that she and Winton "were left holding the sack."[13] Thus, though the "hotbed" (Curtis's term) of anti-nurse anesthetist activity was in Southern California, that group disbanded and transferred the state organization north to San Francisco, where several nurse anesthetists continued to hold meetings. The California State Association of Nurse Anesthetists became an "official" affiliate of the National Association of Nurse Anesthetists in 1935, with its constitution and bylaws modeled on those of the National group. Not surprisingly, Eva Wilson, who had been threatened by the 1928 resolution of the State Board of Medical Examiners, was a member of its Committee on Membership.[14]

In the meantime, Curtis's attorney, McFadden, in January 1931, queried the Attorney General as to whether that office had "ever rendered a legal opinion to the State Medical Board to the effect that the giving of an anesthetic by an unlicensed person was a violation of the Medical Practice Act."[15] The response was quick in coming: no, it had not.

It was the State Board of Medical Examiners that next queried the Attorney General. Charles B. Pinkham, its secretary-treasurer, wrote on August 29, 1933, for an opinion on the interpretation of the law as given by its own legal counsellors, i.e., "to the effect that the administration of anaesthetics by lay persons constituted violations of Section 17 of the Medical Practice Act."[16] The response from U. S. Webb, the Attorney General, on September 26, 1933, began by noting the specific questions posed:

(1) whether a registered nurse may administer anaesthetics for general surgical procedure in a hospital; (2) may a registered nurse administer anaesthetics in the office of a physician and surgeon for minor work; (3) may a registered nurse administer anaesthetics in homes for obstetric cases. Your preface to each question is that the administration of such anaesthetics shall always be under the supervision of the attending physician and surgeon.[17]

The opinion of the Attorney General, rendered in response to the above inquiry, cited the precedent of the *Frank v. South* case in which the Supreme Court of Kentucky, in 1917,

directly held that a nurse who complied with all the requirements of the statutes relative to graduate or trained nurses, did not purport to engage in the practice of medicine, did not have a medical license and administered anaesthetics pursuant to the direction of her medical employer, did not have an office or announce to the public her readiness to treat the sick or afflicted and had never prescribed for anyone, was not engaged in the practice of medicine within the meaning of the Kentucky law.[18]

The opinion then noted that the *Frank v. South* case *did* take into account the fact that the "nurse's own judgment" was involved in the above practice:

> The Supreme Court noted the analogy between the right of a nurse to administer to a patient, medicines prescribed by a physician, even though the administration thereof necessitated the use of the nurse's own judgment and the right of a nurse to give an anaesthetic pursuant to the supervision and direction of a physician. It was pointed out that in neither instance did a nurse attempt to make a diagnosis of the symptoms of the patient, determine the ailment and decide the remedy.[19]

Interestingly, this new opinion noted three major factors in the *Frank v. South* decision favoring the rights of nurse anesthetists: first, "the fact that at the Mayo Clinic where up to 1917 [the date of the Kentucky case] one hundred thousand surgical operations had been performed, anaesthetics were invariably administered by trained nurses," and, second, "that some of the medical associations and organizations of physicians and surgeons in the United States approved the employment of graduate or trained nurses to administer anaesthetics to their patients and some did not."[20] Thus, it was, and would continue to be, the *documented* performance record of nurse anesthetists and the division of opinion within the medical community itself that would provide the essential support to the nurse anesthetists' right to continue their work. There is then cited a third factor: the practice of *nursing*.

Attorney General Webb continues by noting that there was no legal support for the position that the mere fact of being a physician conferred an expertise in the administration of anesthetics:

> In Spain v. Burch, (Mo.) 154 S.W. 172, the court pointed out that "The skill and proficiency by which a physician administering an anaesthetic is to be judged is not to be measured by the usual and ordinary skill possessed by other physicians only, but extends to that possessed by other persons, whose occupation and study gives them an equal or better knowledge of the right methods of its use than is possessed by a general practitioner of medicine."

The latter expression would seem to indicate that the courts of

Missouri have recognized that persons other than physicians might be more skilled in the use of anaesthetics than are physicians. Such seems to be the growing trend of authority.[21]

This opinion concludes by once again citing the *Frank v. South* case, and points to the other factor supporting the nurse anesthetist position: in administering anesthetics, the *nurse* anesthetist functioned as "the physician's hand," that is, functioned as a *nurse*.

In spite of the opinion, the following month the Anesthetic Section of the Los Angeles County Medical Association asked a physician, Dr. William V. Chalmers-Francis, to test legally the right of nurse anesthetists to administer anesthesia. The ironic dimension was intensified by the fact that the nurse anesthetist targeted was one who was a graduate nurse of St. Mary's Hospital School of Nursing, Rochester, Minnesota, who had been giving anesthetics at the Mayo Clinic for the previous ten years.

Dr. Verne C. Hunt, formerly of Mayo Clinic, then surgeon at St. Vincent's Hospital, Los Angeles, invited Dagmar Nelson to come from Minnesota to California to work at the hospital as an anesthetist, to be available to any surgeon who wished her services, but giving Hunt's cases priority. Nelson agreed, although she had been warned by Hunt of the hostility in the area to nurse anesthetists. According to Adeline Curtis, it was the death from asphyxiation of one of his patients—a twenty-three-year-old undergoing minor surgery—that determined Hunt to bring in Nelson rather than continue with practitioners such as the one involved in this unhappy case, a young man with little experience in anesthesia.[22] In a letter of October 27, 1933, to Benjamin W. Black, medical director of Highland Hospital (discussed above), Hunt indicated that the test case was, for him, not an unwelcome event: "This case, of course, will be a test of the State Medical Practice Act, and I hope out of that we will learn what the true practice of medicine might be."[23] This surgeon would devote much energy and money to putting together the strongest possible case for the place of nurse anesthetists in the field—a financial burden that the opposing side would, in spite of all its rhetoric, be reluctant to bear.

The physician anesthetists first sought an injunction to restrain permanently Dagmar Nelson from administering anesthetics. The plaintiffs in this action were Drs. William V. Chalmers-Francis, William Dewey Wightman, and George P. Waller, Jr., along with the Anesthesia Section of the Los Angeles County Medical Association. Nelson's attorneys, the firm of Mott, Vallée and Grant (retained by Hunt and St. Vincent's Hospital) responded on a demurrer, arguing that an injunction was improper, since "plaintiffs are not confronted with an invasion of any of their property rights." Moreover, the demurrer questioned the right of the "so-called Anesthesia Section of the Los Angeles Medical Association" to be party to the suit.[24] Judge Roth of the Superior Court held on March 26, 1934, that while individual physicians might sue to prevent the "unlicensed" from practicing medicine and surgery, the Anesthesia Section had no such right.

It is interesting that *The Bulletin of the Los Angeles County Medical Association* quickly reported in its April 19, 1934, issue, that Judge Roth had enjoined Dagmar Nelson from "so practicing medicine until she has obtained a state license to practice medicine." Nelson's attorneys demanded a retraction from the *Bulletin,* saying: "The article in your Bulletin is so at variance with the true facts it is impossible to understand its publication. One reading it could not escape the conclusion that Miss Nelson was not only illegally practicing medicine, but that such fact had been judicially determined. Likewise the conclusion that St. Vincent's Hospital had been enjoined from illegal acts would be unescapable."[25] The complete retraction appeared in *The Bulletin of the Los Angeles County Medical Association,* noting that, "The information in the exact wording in which it appeared in the Bulletin was sent to the Editor's Desk from what appeared to be an authentic source."[26] The author of that report remains unknown, but the language and argument are familiar.

On July 12, 1934, in the Superior Court of Los Angeles, Judge Allen B. Campbell presiding, Dagmar Nelson went on trial for violating the California Medical Practice Act: practicing medicine without a license. The plaintiffs through their lawyers—LeRoy Anderson and F. L. Kostlan—made it clear that there was nothing personal in this legal action: "We brought this suit on behalf of ourselves and other physicians similarly situated and are naturally not disposed to go after the defendant in this particular case. It is a test question as far as we are concerned. We want to establish, if we can, that . . . the giving of anesthetics and the employment of nurses or any other person who is not a registered physician and surgeon, is in violation of the California Medical Practice Act."[27] The physician-anesthetist argument was that the administration of anesthetics was, in effect, the practice of medicine for the following reasons: "(1) that the surgeon, being separated from the anesthetist by a screen, could in no way supervise the actual administration of an anesthetic; (2) that an anesthetic was a drug, that in administering the drug the anesthetist used his own judgment as to the amount and that in so doing he was treating the patient; (3) that in observing the signs of anesthesia and acting as those signs indicated he should, he was making a diagnosis of the patient's condition."[28]

Not surprisingly, just as the chief witnesses for the plaintiffs were physician anesthetists, the defense depended chiefly on the testimony of surgeons. The defense argument was: "(1) the giving of drugs upon direct or *understood* instruction of a physician was a recognized practice and within the limits of the definition of nursing, (2) that the recognition and the reporting of changes in a patient's condition and acting accordingly under the direct or *understood* supervision of a physician was within the province of nursing, (3) that nursing education as accepted by law gave instruction in the administration of anesthetics and the recognition of the signs and stages of anesthesia and (4) that it was an established practice within the law for registered nurses to give anesthetics as a nursing duty."[29] Ironically, Hodgins's quarrel with nursing notwithstanding, the defense repeatedly argued that anesthesia was within the province of *nursing*.

The twelve-day trial ended on July 27, 1934. The judgment followed shortly:

The above-entitled case having been regularly tried, argued and submitted for decision and the court, being fully advised in the premises, finds:

I. That at the times mentioned in the complaint defendant Nelson was engaged as a nurse anesthetist under the direction and supervision of operating surgeons, and with the knowledge of defendant, St. Vincent's Hospital, a corporation.

II. That the acts of the defendant Nelson under the evidence introduced in this case, do not constitute practicing medicine or surgery under the Medical Practice Act.

III. That the evidence in this case is insufficient to make out a case against defendants, or either of them, of practicing medicine without a license in violation of the Medical Practice Act.

Defendants' motion to strike all the evidence heretofore submitted is denied.

Judgment is ordered for defendants.

Defendants to prepare findings and judgment.

Dated: July 31, 1934

(signed) Allen B. Campbell
Judge[30]

The physician anesthetists decided to appeal the decision, and therefore wrote to members of the Los Angeles County Medical Association requesting financial support of the continued legal action:

The case has been appealed to the higher Courts and this entails heavy costs of somewhere between $1500 and $2000. Dr. Francis has stood most of the work and costs up to date, and we feel that it is a matter worthy of the profession getting behind Dr. Francis. . . .

Please mail a check—as you feel you can to help Dr. Chalmers—Francis . . . and a receipt will be returned for your files, as soon as possible.

We are,

Yours very truly,
Dr. Geo. Waller, Chairman
Dr. James C. Doyle, Sec.
Dr. Arthur Guedel
Dr. C. F. McCuskey
Dr. J. M. Klein,
Committee of Publicity[31]

The haughtiness of propaganda faded with the financial realities of the legal action.

The judgment was upheld by the Supreme Court of California. Its decision, on May 18, 1936, found that Nelson's activities were part of "established and uniformly accepted practice followed by surgeons and nurses." The Supreme Court found this practice "beyond dispute" because of the consideration of "the evidence of the many surgeons who supported the contention of the defendant nurse, and whose qualifications to testify concerning the practice of medicine in this community and elsewhere were established beyond dispute." In addition, previously decided cases (including *Frank v. South*) were "in accord."[32]

In a sense, it was Chalmers-Francis who was "left holding the sack," as Adeline Curtis would say. The request for financial support from fellow physicians was denied:

The regular monthly meeting of the Board of Trustees was held Thursday, August 13 [1936]. . . . A letter from the Anesthesia Section signed by Doctor Charles F. McCuskey, Secretary, was read. The request for financial aid in the payment of attorneys' fees that arose in the test case on the question of nurse anesthetists, upon motion duly made and seconded, was refused.[33]

But Chalmers-Francis's spirit was undaunted. In January 1937, less than one year of the close of the Nelson case, he published the following letter in *Medical Economics:*

More power to Dr. F. H. McMechan.

He has covered with clarity the problem of anesthesia in the United States where technicians have been permitted to develop unrestricted by organized medical authorities. The latter, by their soporific indifference, repeat their historic neglect of the invasion of osteopathy in the field of health work in this country.

Anesthesia is the treatment of painful injury; it calls for prescribing dosages of lethal and dangerous drugs; its successful administration depends on diagnosing the reaction of each patient to the lethal drug to be employed. Treatment, prescription, and diagnosis have, by legal decisions and moral understanding, been ruled as the practice of medicine. Why, therefore, in the United States has the invasion of technicians into the field of anesthesia been permitted? Because there are those who court success by commercializing their profession. The money earned by technicians goes to the treasuries of their employers. Thus, our rights as medical men suffer from vicious invasion for the sake of financial reward.

We must recapture our control of anesthesia. We can do so if we take a lesson from the British Medical Association and organized medicine in Canada. They have protected their respective populations from lowered standards.[34]

Chalmers-Francis here signs himself with the title "President, Associated Anesthetists of the United States and Canada."

A very different tone is taken in Dr. Hunt's address to the Mid-South Postgraduate Nurse Anesthetists' Assembly in Memphis in February 1941. In that speech, he modestly observed, "I believe that as I may have had something to do with maintaining and enhancing the status of nurse anesthetists, they have likewise had much to do with rearing me surgically, for which I continue to feel grateful."[35]

In October of that year, Hunt wrote to Helen Lamb: "Miss Dagmar Nelson, who has given my anesthetics for years, is making a trip to the midwest and I have asked her to include St. Louis and spend a bit of time with you. I am very desirous of having her meet you and see your work."[36] Nelson, Lamb, and Hunt did correspond, with Lamb warmly assuring Hunt that the visit would be made "as interesting as possible" for Nelson: "I feel most flattered that you have asked Miss Nelson to visit our clinic. . . . I will advise Dr. Graham that she is to be here, and if he is in the city I know he will do one of his lobectomies or pneumectomies for her, if she would be interested."[37]

Apparently the relationships were cordial, for Nelson appeared on the membership list of the American Association of Nurse Anesthetists in 1942. In 1944, Dagmar Nelson presented the Association with the transcript of her trial for placement in its Archives.[38]

As was noted, the Nelson case was fought by Dr. Hunt, and supported by fellow surgeons and by California nurse anesthetists such as Adeline Curtis and Sophie Gran Winton. Though the National Association of Nurse Anesthetists did file a brief in amicus curiae for the Supreme Court appeal, its involvement was minimal. The case was a watershed in deciding the legality of nurse anesthesia, but Cleveland was a long way from Los Angeles in the early 1930s, and the young National Association—faced with the illness of Hodgins and few supporting resources—seemed removed from what proved to be the life and death legal struggle unfolding in California. Its major concern was the equally critical matter of its education program.

"My Chief Interest Is in Education."

—Agatha Hodgins, June 20, 1932[39]

It will be recalled that when the Lakeside Hospital Unit, Base Hospital 4, returned to the front after the United States entered the war in 1917, Hodgins did not accompany it. Rather, she contributed by remaining in Cleveland to continue the direction of the Hospital's School of Anesthesia, training nurses, physicians, and dentists. It will also be recalled that, on February 15, 1932, in her letter to Marie Louis of the American Nurses' Association, Hodgins indicated that the need for establishing uniform and stringent criteria for the education of nurse anesthetists was the motive behind her drive for national organization:

> You are doubtless aware that nurses with little or no education on the subject practicing anesthesia, is a serious cause of complex and disturbing difficulties constantly arising. This situation can only be cleared up by our ability to create a classification insuring protection to all concerned. Thus, briefly outlined, are the reasons leading to the organization.[40]

When, four months later, she corresponded with Adeline Curtis regarding matters of professional organization, Hodgins noted that her own plans were to contribute to the Association's future through development of its education program: "Although I am very willing indeed to do what I can in regard to the organization, my chief interest is in education and I do not feel that I would be able to accept responsibility of this sort for a long period of time."[41] Perhaps she had a sense of her deteriorating health, for six months later she suffered a heart attack and was forced into semiretirement. She would, however, not simply keep a vigilant eye on the Association's education program, but would play a role in shaping it.

There were others who were interested in standardizing nurse anesthetist education and establishing a national certification examination. When Gertrude Fife addressed the first national convention of the National Association of Nurse Anesthetists in 1933, she called for a committee to investigate nurse anesthesia schools for the purpose of accreditation and for a national board examination for nurse anesthetists. These steps, she said, would "safeguard the surgeon's interest, the interest of the hospitals, and the interest of the public."[42] What was not known at the time—intentionally—was the role that physicians had in shaping the plan that would accelerate the professionalization of nurse anesthetists. Fife told the rest of the story in a 1971 memoir, saying, "no record would be complete unless the examination program were included."[43]

> One day Dr. Lenhart [of University Hospitals, Cleveland] came into the operating room and said, "I have been thinking about your Association, and I may have an idea. Come into my office and we will discuss it." When I got there, he was sitting in his big chair, with his feet up, chewing a cigar and looking into space. He said Dr. Howard Karsner had been involved in starting the National Board of Examinations for doctors and he wondered if such a program could be worked out for our group. He said he would like to have me discuss the possibility with Dr. Karsner.

Fife was taken aback and "apprehensive," for though the "Great Dr. Karsner"—Professor of Pathology at Western Reserve University—"was held in high esteem, [she] had heard how difficult he could be," and the prospect of an interview with him was, she said, "unthinkable." Reassured by Lenhart, Fife met with Karsner. She recalled that the first conference was brief, she stating "the case" in the fewest possible words, and Karsner asking a couple of questions, concluding with "You will hear from me." And so she did. Back in Karsner's office two days later, he

> handed me two full pages of instructions. He had outlined in detail the steps to be taken, how to sell it to the Education Committee; also how the examination should be conducted, etc. He even included questions that would be brought up against such a program and the answers to some.

The delicacy of the matter was not lost on Karsner. He had further advice for Fife:

He said he wanted me to study it, memorize the steps, put it down in my own words and use it as my contribution. He said it would lose its effectiveness if it were not presented as coming from within our group. He said, "I have given you the tools—you use them and come to me for consultation."

An interesting sidelight on Fife's relationship with the "Great Dr. Karsner" is provided in Fife's observation that

> I became very fond of Dr. Karsner. His keen mind could cut through details and pinpoint the real issue and if he didn't have a solution, he was honest enough to say so. He was intolerant of indecision and evasiveness. With him, something was right or it was wrong. (Later I gave Dr. Karsner an anesthetic for manipulation of his shoulder.)[44]

But gaining acceptance for the plan of a national examination and accreditation of schools was not easy, chiefly because Hodgins favored another approach to establishing the position of the professional nurse anesthetist: state registration. Her reasons for doing so may have been the result of her conviction that the work fell under neither the category of medicine nor of nursing, and that nurse anesthetists needed the protection of a separate legal status. She may also have been affected by years of listening to the charge leveled by physician-anesthetists hostile to the existence of nurses in the field, that they were "unlicensed" practitioners.

As mentioned above, Hodgins was "forced" into semiretirement, first by the heart attack that kept her hospitalized for six months, then by her own physicians, and finally by the administration of Lakeside Hospital. Fife recalled that, even during Hodgins's hospital stay, she "was going to run the department from her room," having Fife bring reports to her. Hodgins's doctors finally gave orders that the coronary patient was to have no visitors. Leaving the hospital for her home on Cape Cod, Hodgins continued to be concerned about the Association's education program, writing letters in a small, neat hand, that were "miles long," sent in packages, and always about the same thing: education.

After a few months' stay on the Cape, Hodgins returned to Lakeside Hospital. Said Fife, "Nobody knew. All of a sudden she showed up. Comes up to the office and takes charge, . . . sits right down, as if she'd never been away, as if nothing had ever happened." It was left to Dr. R. H. Bishop, Director of the hospital, to make clear to her that, because of her heart condition, she *was* retired. (Her reaction would prefigure that of a later, powerful Association leader,

Florence McQuillen, when different conditions forced her into retirement.) Fife recalled of Hodgins that

> They retired her on a good pension and she didn't have to worry, but she didn't want it. . . . It made it awfully hard for us. . . . She blamed everybody.[45]

She also continued to work for state registration of nurse anesthetists as the desired path to standardizing their education.

Fife also continued *her* lobbying campaign, favoring the goal of a uniform education program achieved through the accreditation of schools and a national examination. In a speech on February 14, 1934, she addressed all of these issues. The matter of standardizing the education program was urgent because of the existence of inferior schools, those whose programs were too brief, or were limited to practical training only. Fife noted that this latter method "makes practical anesthetists only, and *our educational methods discouraged and condemned many years ago the practice of 'learning by doing.'*" She added, "Fortunately these schools are in the great minority." (emphasis added)

On the matter of accreditation, Fife said:

> Our problem now as I see it is to work for the standardization of schools. . . . The Association will serve as a pace-maker for the better schools and will influence the poorer schools to meet the required standards. The Association will secure for schools on its list a recognition throughout the United States such as could not be secured in any other way, and will make possible the acceptance of guiding principles in matters pertaining to the education of the nurse anesthetist. Indeed, the recognition of a school will serve as a guarantee of the institution's efficiency, and the high standards thus established will make individual membership in the National Association a distinctive honor and a guarantee of her good standing in the field of anesthesia.

Regarding the matter of a national examination, Fife stressed its *practical* advantages over that of state registration:

> Furthermore, every anesthetist should be required to pass National Board examinations. I do not believe that state board registration for nurse anesthetists is either practical or possible. Quicker and more direct action can be obtained through a National Board, and more uniform methods of teaching will result from the establishment of universal rather than sectional standards. The examining

board should be chosen by the National Association and should be responsible for the preparation of the examinations, the arrangements necessary for the examinations—to be taken within the states—and responsible for the final decision which would permit the National Association to grant a certificate to those having successfully passed the examinations.[46]

The exchange of letters between Hodgins and Fife in August and September of 1934 reveals not only a discussion of the issues, but a contest of wills. Though Fife later said of Hodgins that "Miss Hodgins was Miss Hodgins, . . . and you didn't press"; "She would have her way. She was determined . . . and you just got out of the way."[47] Fife stood her ground, once again stressing the impracticality of a state registration drive.

Hodgins's "determination" is clearly apparent in her letter to Fife of August 23, 1934:

I have, as you remember, emphasized to you and others, but most particularly to you last January as President of our Association, the necessity of instituting steps to prepare the way for National registration and securing if necessary legislation to make effective and well defined the status of the Nurse Anesthetists throughout the country. In a later discussion this spring, your reply to my repeated suggestion for action on this matter was that agitations against the Nurse Anesthetists were not likely to prove serious and that the Hospital Association was watching legislation. You also stressed the expense of legislation. It would seem from what has occurred in Indiana that this was perhaps too optimistic a viewpoint. I am therefore reiterating in this letter my conviction that unless we make secure our status by registration, we are building on an insecure foundation and the fine work the Association has accomplished in other directions may come to nought. . . . In regard to expense, this must be met by assessing the members.[48]

Fife's response on August 29, 1934, emphasized just *how* expensive Hodgins's plan would be (and how strategically risky, as the physician-anesthetists would find out when they lost the Nelson case):

Relative to National Registration for nurse anesthetist, it is my understanding that national registration could not be obtained unless it were first passed by the legislatures in the individual states. The approximate cost to prepare a bill to be presented in the legislature is about $500. In addition to this we should have about $200 available for lobbying purposes. As I see it, we might be able to finance any proposed legislation in one or two states, but an intensive program in this direction would prove prohibitive from the financial standpoint. It is also a question in my mind whether it is wise to start any legislation at this time. If we were defeated in even one state the result would undoubtedly be disastrous for the entire country.[49]

The financial burden of a state registration effort made even Hodgins rethink the matter. (The puzzlement expressed at the end of her reply to Fife's letter is reminiscent of Hodgins's somewhat bewildered reaction to the American Nurses' Association's response to her 1931 proposal for affiliation.) On September 15, 1934, Hodgins wrote:

> The figures given in your fifth paragraph would certainly make National Registration by such means prohibitive. I had no idea lobbying was so lucrative a job. Surely there must be a way out—more practical and within our means.
>
> In stressing the fact that we should institute steps to prepare the way for registration, I did not intend to imply that any precipitate action should be taken at this critical time. In states where opposition is active we can only meet the situation by our ability to refute the opposition, in presenting a record of fine service rendered the country at large by the nurse anesthetist. . . .
>
> I remember quite distinctly discussing with you the question of the "National Board of Examiners." At that time the information you had was a bit indefinite, and I am delighted that further study now reveals it as a possible solution of our problem for securing National registration. . . . Applied to our own case, although we do create a National Board of Examiners and require all anesthetists to pass the examinations required by the same, their legal right to practice depends on the acceptance by the State Board of Medical Examiners, in each particular state, of the certificate granted the candidate by our "National Board of Examiners." So somehow or other we must come back to state registration. . . .
>
> While I can quite understand that such a body as the "National Board of Examiners" could be created and function, without legislative sanction, I cannot see how registration can be obtained, except through a body legally authorized to grant it. We will all agree that until registration is obtained, we have no assurance of security in being able to practice our profession. . . .
>
> The crux of the situation is, how long is it safe to wait without making an effort to consolidate our position by working for regis-

tration, preferably in a state favorably inclined to nurse anesthetists and in which no active opposition has been in evidence?[50]

With very limited financial resources, and with the need to depend on the volunteer efforts of full-time nurse anesthetists, the implementation of association goals understandably proceeded slowly. The minimum standards for the schools of nurse anesthesia accepted by the association trustees at its first national meeting in 1933 were revised in 1935, and again in 1936. It was at that fourth annual meeting, in Cleveland, that a "Recommended Curriculum" was adopted and published in full in the May 1937 issue of *The Bulletin of the National Association of Nurse Anesthetists* as the "Revised Report of the Educational Committee: Recommendations Regarding Schools of Anesthesia for Nurses." The lengthy and thorough document (the work of Chairman Helen Lamb and her Committee, Olive L. Berger, Mae B. Cameron, Mabel Hard, and Mary H. Muller) recommended, in brief, that

> Schools of Anesthesia, whose graduates are to merit highest rating by the National Association of Nurse Anesthetists, give to their students *a training both theoretical and practical* which is equivalent to the curriculum above set forth in this report; and that minimal standards be:
>
> Length of course—six months (with one year advocated)
>
> Hours of recorded "class room instruction"—95
>
> Hours of recorded "operating room class instruction"—18
>
> Number of cases administered—325
>
> Of this accredited 325, at least 250 must be general surgical; 25 should be obstetrical; 25 may be dental; 25 may be divided between spinals, locals, et cetera.[51] (emphasis added)

The matter of inspection of schools was being seen more and more as not then feasible, given the lack of funds to staff the enterprise and a concern for potential legal problems that might arise from challenging the legitimacy of a particular school of nurse anesthesia.

In September 1935 Fife wrote to the association's Board of Trustees, presenting a practical plan for the implementation of a national examination:

> If the National organization appointed say seven people on an examining board, including possibly two or three outstanding sur-

geons (the details of which could be worked out later) to prepare examination questions periodically, to be given to every student before graduation from any School of Anesthesia that wished to be recognized by the National, we at least would be able to make certain that the members of the National organization were qualified. Someone within the state who is not connected with the school could act for the Examining Board in seeing that the examination was conducted in an ethical manner. A certificate similar to State Board certificates could be awarded to the applicant passing the examination.[52]

Fife was correct in her prediction that "in a few years the superintendents and surgeons generally would require their anesthetists to be recognized by the National Association. After all, the superintendents and surgeons are not interested in whether the examining board has obtained legislative sanction—they are interested in making certain that their anesthetists are equipped to give anesthetics."[53]

Fife's position was embraced at the 1936 national convention, in part, probably because, as the Education Committee reported, there was now a "definite trend in the direction of National Boards of Examinations by various professional groups, as noted by the recently created American Board of Surgery (for national examination and certification of general surgeons), and also the Council on Dental Education, organized only two months ago 'for the examination and listing of (dental) specialists.' A carefully worked out plan looking forward to eventual national examination and certification for nurse anesthetists would therefore seem to be *peculiarly* in keeping with the current trend of professional thought in our fields."[54] (emphasis added) But, as Fife knew—and was pledged to keep secret—there was nothing "peculiar" at all about this nurse specialty group being in the forefront of this trend: Drs. Lenhart and Karsner had directed them there.

A Question of "Happy Relationships"

Still another recommendation of Lamb's Education Committee in its 1936 report led to an intriguing—and still cloudy—incident that might have brought about an alliance between nurse anesthetists and physician anesthetists. The Education Committee saw the need for the Association to involve a major surgical or hospital group in its plans to certify the capability of its members:

With that thought in mind, and giving heed to the growing feeling that the whole future of the nurse anesthetist and the conditions under which she is to function are likely to be intimately related to affiliation with, and endorsement by, the great National surgical and hospital groups, this Committee feels that it becomes incumbent upon our Association to prepare for presentation to such groups a concrete program which will set forth not only the standard of education and training which a nurse anesthetist is expected to have achieved, but also at the same time furnish it with a working plan for demonstrating whether or not an applicant for certification does possess that knowledge and has acquired the requisite training.[55]

In her 1937 Education Committee Report, Lamb said that "[We] have contacted individual members of the American Board of Surgery and of the American Hospital Association and have received favorable reaction to the idea behind the plan, without under-rating the many problems to be overcome in working out the details practically."[56] It is worth noting that Lamb's contact on the American Board of Surgery was her associate from Barnes Hospital, St. Louis, Dr. Evarts Graham, for whom she acted as anesthetist. It helps explain her great confidence in that agency.

The "problems" Lamb referred to were, in fact, considerable—finally proving insurmountable. Efforts by the American Board of Surgery to affect a positive relationship between the National Association of Nurse Anesthetists and the American Board of Anesthesiology were resented by the latter group. It had been newly formed (1937) and was operating under its "parent," the American Board of Surgery. In a study published in 1982, Dr. Frederick P. Haugen presented the following description of events:

Minutes of later meetings in 1938 disclosed a growing feeling that the Board of Surgery was pressuring the Board of Anesthesia to embrace the national organization of nurse anesthetists and to put the two groups into "happy relationships." *It was pointed out that no other specialty board was functioning as a supervisor of the training of technicians* and the Board of Anesthesia was convinced that it should not become involved in the matter. During the formative meetings of the Board, representatives of the American Board of Surgery met with it: the relationship was irksome because of the differences in viewpoint.[57] (emphasis added)

Rosemary Stevens, who, like Haugen, had access to the minutes of the American Board of Anesthesiology, added another dimension to the discussion in her major study, *American Medicine and the Public Interest:*

The nurses, seeking their own program of certification, made over-
tures to the American Board of Anesthesiology in 1938 *which might
have enabled the two movements to combine and the anesthesiologists* [as
physician-anesthetists now called themselves] *to take on responsibility
for the nurses' training.* But the attitude of hostility was already set,
and the nurses were summarily rejected; indeed, there was anxiety
(probably not unfounded at the time) that if the board approved
training schools for nurse anesthetists, surgeons would feel they
had a carte blanche to replace their medical anesthesiologists with
nurses. (emphasis added)

Stevens's concluding observation was one not lost on the nurse anesthetists of 1938:

In so doing the board missed a golden opportunity, for nurse
anesthetists were increasingly demanded by the hospitals.[58]

But: if the young American Board of Anesthesiology was concerned
about *establishing* its independence from the American Board of Surgery, the National Association of Nurse Anesthetists was equally concerned about *maintaining* its independence—especially in its
educational programs. At its board meeting in New York on November 26, 1938, the day before there was to be a meeting with members
of the American Board of Surgery and the American Board of Anesthesiology, President Miriam Shupp reported to the board that she
was not informed about the agenda for the joint meeting. When
Lamb joined the group later in the session, she explained that her
"reaction was that this is merely a contact meeting. It will be discussed
with their own particular group, our own particular group and the
Board of our Association before any agreement will be entered into."
Lamb repeated that the "situation arose very quickly," and that "It was
a surprise to me that this meeting was held so quickly."[59]

Years later, Shupp would recall the incident and her own feelings
on the matter of "affiliation":

Helen Lamb and I had a difference of opinion on this. She thought
we'd be better off to hook up with the surgeons—of course the
A.N.A. was out—but Helen was of the opinion that we'd be better
off at the American Board of Surgery. At that time the anesthesiologists were sort of a subsidiary group of the surgeons. But I
didn't trust the Boards and I didn't trust all the surgeons, and I felt
that for the time being we'd be better sticking with the American
Hospital Association, where we knew we had backing. Of course we
argued pro and con, and I said I wouldn't vote for them. I wouldn't

vote for any hook up with the surgeons at that time. Then we got ourselves enmeshed with them and then found out that we were under the anesthesiologists. Well, I just didn't trust the anesthesiologists, and I thought the surgeons might be dupes because they listened to the anesthesiologists. So I said no way would I vote for that, so they tabled it and we stayed with the American Hospital Association.[60]

Fife, who was also present at the November 25, 1938, board meeting later recalled that, when Hodgins got "wind" of the gathering, she hurried to New York from Cape Cod, to "bust in on it." While the minutes note Hodgins in attendance, no words are recorded. But Fife recalled her as one who "saved the day."[61]

The Department of Education

In May 1940 Hodgins, now a member of the Committee on Education (Lamb remained Chairman), announced in the *Bulletin of the American Association of Nurse Anesthetists* a new "Department of Education," representing "the educational teaching program" of the Association. Noting that an "inclusive curriculum" had already been published, and a survey of schools was being undertaken "to obtain firsthand information as to the educational facilities of the same," Hodgins told of a new plan whereby the *Bulletin* would be utilized as a vehicle for standardizing and elevating the education of nurse anesthetists. "The scope of this program will include a series of articles on the physiology of respiration, circulation and nerve function as related to anesthesia. It will also elaborate in teaching articles the educational content of the accepted curriculum."[62] Clearly, Hodgins was extending her concern from that of not only teaching the student nurse anesthetists, but to teaching their teachers:

The function of this program will be threefold; first—that of providing to schools a uniform approach to curricular contents, thus standardizing the education given the student; second—by presentation of current material in teaching form, keep[ing] the education of the student in pace with progress made in anesthesia; third—publication of this teaching material will not only provide continuity of instruction but will make the "Bulletin" still more valuable and permanent as a reference journal on teaching activities. As the value of certain articles, as teaching guides, becomes apparent, it is hoped that such will be re-edited by the Correlating Committee, and reprinted by the Publishing Committee, in more convenient form for use by school instructors.[63]

Hodgins also voiced her hope that, "in due time," the Association would sponsor teacher institutes.

Hodgins's respect for Lamb is evidenced in the fact that, in this same year, Hodgins asked her to accept the presidential candidacy of the Association, adding that she would be willing to take Lamb's place as Chairman of the Committee on Education. Lamb had reservations about doing so, which Hodgins addressed in a letter to her on July 12, 1940. It is an interesting document, revealing the philosophy that drove Hodgins and shaped her life. And there is even warmth in the letter—a quality not many of her contemporaries associated with her:

Chatham, Mass
July 12, 1940

Dear Helen:

Yesterday I received from Miss Shupp your letter to her refusing the candidacy for president of A.A.N.A. also a note asking if I would try and persuade you to reconsider your decision as the Board is unanimous in wanting you.

I had already written asking you to undertake this responsibility, giving as my prime reason, these two factors: your own career and life, and the need of the Association. I am asking now that you do reconsider your decision, because of the unanimous feeling of the Board, that you are the person at this time, most needed as head of the organization.

You said in your letter to Miss Shupp that you were willing to give unstintingly of time and effort, you have proved that: now I am asking you to retranslate that statement into a resolution to take this presidency. I have refrained all my life from asking my friends to do things on my advice, but this once I am asking you, because I think I can see more clearly than you how much the Association needs your forthright courage and sincerity of purpose at this time. I also realize, as perhaps you do not, that if you refuse, your courage will never again be so high in quality or your own discipline of spirit so well controlled, both of these are necessary if you are to keep that firm grasp of life which brings a constant feeling of being part of creation and so really alive, living and happy. This I want you to have, and it can only be freely obtained by venturing to do the things you feel you can't.

As I see it, your duty lies in accepting this candidacy and I have never known you yet to shirk that. So write Miss Shupp and tell her you will allow your name to stand and so make us all happy.

Affectionately,
(signed) Agatha Hodgins[64]

Lamb yielded to Hodgins's persuasion, and served as Association President for two terms, 1940–41 and 1941–42.

It was during 1941 that the survey of schools was finally launched. Unfortunately, so was America's entry into another world war. The concerns of the Association were dramatically affected. Whereas it had been trying to raise and standardize the school programs, it now had the immense task of *maintaining* the ground that had been gained.

Nurse Anesthetist Service in World War II

In September 1940 Beatrice M. Quin, RN, of the Army Nurse Corps, spoke at the annual AANA meeting on "Anesthesia in Army Hospitals." Her speech, which might be viewed as a recruitment exercise with a view to the probable imminent involvement of this country in then still-foreign war, emphasized the progress nurses had made in the Army Nurse Corps: "The year 1920 gave to [Army Nurses] the many privileges and benefits of relative rank, and some years later the nurse was given the right to retire for length of service and also for disability. . . . I think one may say that the nurse anesthetist finally made a very definite place for herself in army hospitals." As for anesthesia education, "a full course of training in this subject is given to members of the Corps at the Army Medical Center, Washington, and also at some of the general hospitals in other parts of the country. Also members of the Corps may be sent for training in anesthesia to various civilian medical centers, and during the period of training receive full salary and allowances. Approximately fifty trained anesthetists are now on active duty at the various army posts."[65]

While Quin went on to point out that army hospitals were located in attractive settings, including Hawaii, "giving the added attraction of travel," and that army nurses also enjoyed "comfortable and attractive living quarters, eight hour duty, the enjoyment of many sports such as riding, swimming, tennis, golf, et cetera, while not forgetting the opportunities for further study," she also had to note a feature that the American Association of Nurse Anesthetists would focus on: "The Corps continues to expand, and at present has a permanent personnel of approximately one thousand nurses. *These nurses are not appointed for assignment to special duties, but any nurse having special training is usually given the opportunity of using this knowledge.*"[66] (emphasis added) It was this lack of assurance that the nurse-anesthetist specialists would in fact serve in their own discipline that caused difficulties for the national Association.

Another concern of the Association was the increase in emergency-training programs in anesthesia that threatened to undermine the hard-won progress made in the Association's educational program:

> During this critical period, your Committee on Education feels that its greatest contribution may lie in defending the important gains that have been heretofore achieved in the standards of our education—encouraging in fullest manner the utilization of our already well-organized and effectively functioning Schools of Anesthesia rather than countenance the draining of inadequately planned new teaching enterprises, whose chief justification only too often lies in merely that particular institution's desire for additional individual staff service.[67]

Finally, there was the problem of maintaining morale among the overworked anesthetists. The situation brought to Miriam Shupp's mind the words of the Red Queen in *Alice in Wonderland:* "Now *here* you see it takes all the running you can do to stay in the same place."[68]

The Association had received many inquiries from members desiring to volunteer for military service. As a result, in September 1940—at the same meeting Quin addressed—Shupp was appointed chairman of a committee to investigate the status of volunteer nurse anesthetists in the military. From Major Julia O. Flikke, Superintendent Army Nursing Corps, she received the following policy statement:

> Nurse Anesthetists are appointed to the Army Nurse Corps in the grade of nurse, with the relative rank of 2nd Lieutenant. They are subject to all the regulations governing regular Army nurses. Since there is a need for anesthetists in the Nurse Corps at present, they are usually assigned to that duty. However, in some of the smaller Army hospitals, where more than one Nurse Anesthetist is on duty, they may be assigned to duties other than those of anesthetist.[69]

From US Navy Rear Admiral Ross T. McIntire, Surgeon General, USN, came the following explanation:

> Under existing Navy Regulations there is no provision whereby nurses may be appointed in the Nurse Corps of the Navy or Naval Reserve for duty limited to the administration of anesthetics. All appointments of nurses are for general nursing duties. However, if a member of the Navy Nurse Corps is qualified in the administration of anesthetics, she may be assigned to that duty by the Commanding Officer of the Naval Hospital or Station to which she is attached.
>
> Modification of the present arrangements is not contemplated. It

is considered to be to the best interests of the Medical Department not to designate nurses for the administration of anesthetics only, but to appoint applicants who hold this qualification as nurses for general nursing duties.[70]

Thus, the following unsigned notice in the August 1941 *Bulletin of the American Association of Nurse Anesthetists* emphasized to Association members that "whether the nurse anesthetist joins the Army or Navy service directly or through the Red cross, she has the status and rank of nurse":

> While in view of the present need for anesthetists she would probably be assigned to duties in anesthesia, she must understand that since there is no separate division in either the Army or Navy for enlistment as merely anesthetist, she must be prepared to accept any assignment in general nursing, in which the service sees fit to place her. To the best of our knowledge, most of those of our members who have already entered the military service in this present emergency, are doing regular ward duty.

The Association, then, made the following recommendation to its members:

> With the critical need before us for supplying more well trained nurse anesthetists to service the acute shortage which exists in civilian hospitals throughout the United States, the American Association of Nurse Anesthetists is reluctant to urge the individuals of this highly trained group to forsake their specialized and badly needed service in these civilian hospitals, for possibly general nursing service in the military forces, under the regulations as they now exist.

Another mode of wartime service was also suggested to members:

> Many of the University centers have organized "hospital units," that are subject to call in emergency. If an anesthetist does not desire to enroll for active service at this time, she can volunteer to the head of such hospital unit for service with it as anesthetist in the event that unit is called into service.[71]

In a signed editorial in the February 1942 *Bulletin of the American Association of Nurse Anesthetists* Gertrude Fife noted that nurse anesthetists throughout the country continued to write the Association, saying they were willing to serve wherever they were most needed. After briefly recapping the service of nurse anesthetists in World War I, Fife observed that the military status of nurse anesthetists "so far as we know at this writing . . . is the same" as had been described some six months earlier. Fife then reminded members that there was a "civilian army" to be served, one "laboring at top speed 'behind the front,' [which] constitutes the first line of the defensive and grand offensive efforts upon which final victory depends." She urged:

> Each anesthetist who remains faithfully at her post of duty assists in developing a high morale among the large population which each . . . institution serves. The industrial worker who knows that in time of illness he and his family will receive the highest type of medical, surgical, and nursing care, will feel free to throw all his energies into the task of helping produce more and still more of the essential materials of which our country and its allies are in urgent need.[72]

In March 1942 AANA President Helen Lamb wrote to the heads of both the Army and Navy Nurse Corps, urging that nurse anesthetists be assigned to anesthesia service and given an appropriate rank. Unlike the replies received from these offices in the autumn of 1940, there is reflected here—especially on the part of Army Colonel Flikke—a greater recognition of the wisdom of using nurse anesthetists in their field of specialty. She replied to Lamb on April 2:

> Acknowledgment is hereby made of your letter of March 16, suggesting appropriate rank for nurse anesthetists. Under existing regulations, all nurses must be appointed in the Corps in the grade of nurse with the relative rank of Second Lieutenant and be available for any assignment in which their services may be required.
>
> During peace time this was a logical provision, since except in the Army General Hospitals the administration of anesthesia was not a full time job, nor has it been possible for us to secure an increase in the Nurse Corps quota to provide nurses for that specific assignment.
>
> However, under existing circumstances it seems quite necessary and highly desirable to secure as great a number of qualified nurse anesthetists as possible for the Army and a recommendation for special emergency regulations to provide for the appointment of qualified nurse anesthetists in an appropriate grade has been forwarded to the Adjutant General. Upon receipt in this office of information concerning the action taken by the War Department on our recommendation, you will be notified concerning the details.[73]

On March 25, Miss Sue M. Dauser, Superintendent of the Navy Nurse Corps, replied:

When a nurse anesthetist requests appointment in the Navy Nurse Corps we endeavor to determine whether or not she is willing to make her services a little more variable than is specifically stated on her application, since in most Naval Hospitals the nurse anesthetist is not continually engaged with anesthesia. Paramount in every Naval Hospital program is supervision and instruction of hospital corpsmen and the nurse anesthetist has an additional detail in dressing room and surgical supervision which entails her share in this instruction. We have found the nurse anesthetist is willing to accept Navy duty on these conditions, since a similar situation exists in many civilian hospitals.

We realize and appreciate the value of nurses with specific educational advantages and we feel that she above all can understand the service situation in which she finds herself and can make adjustments that are satisfactory to all concerned.

As yet we have not found it necessary to detail anesthetists to bedside nursing care and it is doubted if such duty assignment will ever become necessary.[74]

The issue for AANA leaders was *not* whether nurse anesthetists should volunteer for military service, but whether the military would recognize a clinical specialty within nursing, and allow its members to make the greatest use of their training. It would be as though the armed forces were to group all physicians into a single category, with no recognition of their various specializations. But, in fact, the very opposite occurred in the medical corps: this war contributed to and accelerated the specialization of American medicine.[75]

The nurse anesthetists would have to wait until the end of World War II for such recognition. In August 1947 Lieutenant Colonel Katherine E. Baltz, an Educational Consultant with the Army Nurse Corps, published in the *Journal of the American Association of Nurse Anesthetists* an essay titled, "The Value of Special Training in Anesthesia for the Army Nurse." In it she addressed the matter of the underutilization and misassignment of some personnel by describing the awesome complexity of the situation:

During the war, the Army not only had to supplement the supply of nurse anesthetists but also had to make sure that anesthetists were available in all areas in which they were needed. The rapid and efficient transportation of a particular service to a particular area for a particular purpose could not be accomplished overnight. In order to meet military needs, personnel must be procured, equipped, trained, and transported well in advance of the time they are expected to function in their respective capacities. Thousands of nurses had to be assigned to installations in the United States and to hundreds of units that were shipped overseas. Because of the magnitude of the job, one can readily understand why some nurse anesthetists were misassigned. In World War II there may have been more anesthetists than were needed in some places, but nowhere did we fail to have anesthetists when they were needed. If there was a waste of medical facilities, it was an accident of war, the result of having to be prepared everywhere, at every moment, for every type of attack.[76]

A resounding rallying call for both civilian *and* military service on the part of nurse anesthetists was given in an unsigned Editorial in the August 1942 *Bulletin of the American Association of Nurse Anesthetists*— even though there was still not certitude that those in military service would be assigned to anesthesia:

We sincerely hope that an appropriate grade will be granted the anesthetist by the Adjutant General, but whether or not this is possible (bearing in mind that our problem is only one of countless others facing the Adjutant General) this is our war and we as nurse anesthetists must place our services at the disposal of our government and our boys in the Army and Navy must be taken care of. The younger anesthetists must be relieved for duty with the armed forces and the older anesthetists must put their shoulders to the wheel and push nurse anesthetist service to the top with the same invincible spirit that we expect from those who are fighting our battles in far-away lands.[77]

The Diversity of Anesthesia Training in the Military

The Association's additional concern that its educational programs and plans not be compromised was very well-founded. But the demand for nurse anesthetists in both the military and civilian spheres were so great that the Association could not contain the growth of emergency-training programs. But, what it could do—and did with determination, in spite of the added burdens that the war brought— was proceed in developing its programs for a National Examination and School Accreditation.

Baltz traced the history of the army's own nurse anesthesia training program—which necessarily grew shorter and shorter as the war intensified:

> During the war, the ever increasing need for nurse anesthetists required the Army to initiate some program for their training. Approximately 15,000,000 patients were admitted to Army hospitals during the war, and something had to be done to provide the anesthesia service needed for these patients' care. In November, 1943, 432 nurse anesthetists were distributed among some 1,000 medical installations throughout the United States and in overseas theaters. Some of these anesthetists were Army trained, and others were members of the American Association of Nurse Anesthetists who had been appointed to the Army Nurse Corps. With the invasion of the European mainland and the push through the Pacific Islands toward Japan, the need for more trained nurse anesthetists became apparent. Accordingly the Army launched a full blown training program. Between December, 1941, and December, 1945, approximately 600 Army nurses completed courses in anesthesiology in some 55 Army general hospitals throughout the United States. Overseas, abbreviated courses in anesthesiology were given nurses within earshot of battle. Depending on the needs of the service, the course of training in anesthesiology for the Army nurse ranged from three to six months during the war. Although it was originally planned that the courses should be of six months' duration, in many instances the need for anesthetists became so acute that the courses had to be shortened and accelerated. Hospitals were receiving hundreds of casualties needing surgery, and nurse anesthetists had to be put in the field at the earliest possible date. Accordingly, the training program was not what the Army desired or considered sufficient. However, the supervision of the anesthesia service was well controlled, and every nurse anesthetist worked under either a medical officer or a trained nurse anesthetist.[78]

As Baltz (and Quin, above) indicated, some army nurses had received anesthesia training before the war crisis deepened. Edith A. Aynes was one such army nurse, who requested permission from Major Flikke in 1939 to pursue anesthesia training. Aynes was sent to Jewish Hospital, Philadelphia, for six months' training under Hilda Salomon. Aynes later recalled her experience:

> The school was under the medical jurisdiction of a non-anesthesiologist, but the responsibility for the school was in the

hands of Hilda Salomon, a nurse who had given thousands of general anesthetics without an anesthetic death. She was a small, dignified, unruffled, efficient woman who would have remained calm in the middle of an atomic attack, especially if patients were involved.

To be certain that we had learned the difference between the nurse's duty as anesthetist and the surgical nurse's job, we were absolutely forbidden to function surgically in *any* way in the operating room—not even to tie the surgeon's gown. Our clear responsibility was the *patient*, and the patient only.

The prohibition on surgical activity for the student anesthetists was issued by Miss Salomon and not by the surgical supervisor because scrub nurses, under pressure from the surgeons, issued too many orders to the students. Since every student anesthetist had *been* an operating-room nurse at one time or another, if only during training, it was difficult to sit on a stool at the head of the table with a patient under spinal or local anesthesia and see a surgical nurse waiting impatiently for someone to tie the strings of her sterile gown before she could set up for a surgeon who was breathing down her back. Nevertheless, the rule was strictly enforced. "The patient," Miss Salomon said, "was not to be abandoned!"

Interns and residents gave very few anesthetics at Jewish Hospital, but they were required to have experience with a few during their internships in order to familiarize themselves with the agents used. In 1939, we used chloroform, ether, nitrous oxide, avertin (a rectal anesthesia), a couple of intravenous anesthetics, and nitrous oxide and ether in combination. A gas called cyclopropane had just come on the market, but it was taught in relatively few schools. The Surgeon General said that we did not need to learn to administer it because it was too dangerous for the Army's personnel since enlisted men and nurses were often drafted at a moment's notice to give "a few whiffs."[79]

Aynes's future with the Army Nurse Corps, however, was not to be in anesthesia, but in the new Public Relations Department of the Office of the Surgeon General.

Gertrude Fife, like Hilda Salomon, received anesthesia students from both the army and navy at her school at Lakeside Hospital, Cleveland. Years later, she was asked: "What was it like running an anesthesia department during World War II?" Fife replied with characteristic simplicity: "It was rough."

She went on to explain: "It was rough from this standpoint. You were understaffed. The student body was overcrowded. You had all kinds of people being sent to you. We had no control over the people from the army or navy. Fortunately they sent good people, but they weren't used to working as hard as we were. But you carried them through just the same. And we had great cooperation from the army. One time they sent a couple of men to investigate, and they went back satisfied that we were giving good training."[80]

Barbara Draper was an army nurse given wartime training while stationed in an English hospital in 1943. Having had two years of college before entering a three-year RN program at Children's Hospital, Denver, Draper's academic background was more sophisticated than many of her fellow nurses. It led her into anesthesia:

> One day the chief nurse came to me and said I had been chosen to become an anesthetist because I had had chemistry and biology in college. I was delighted, but scared of this new assignment. For one month four of us met with a physician who taught us anesthesia techniques, and more about respiratory systems, cardiac, b/P, and pentothal.
>
> Most of the cases involved imbedded pieces of shrapnel. We prepped the patient and then the surgeon would say, "Give the pentothal." The scrub nurse was a man and he would hang onto the arm or leg and we would give 20 cc's of pentothal. As the patient dropped to his lowest point, the surgeon would cut, and start looking for the foreign body. If the patient moved, we gave more pentothal. I think they used a little local, too, if it took very long. The repeated 2 cc's or 4 cc's of pentothal would hold the patient until we sewed him up.
>
> There was a gas machine of sorts that could be brought out if we got into trouble, but the patients were all young, healthy men, and the doctor walked between the four of us, sort of standing by if we did something wrong. I can remember getting called down to a ward because some post-op patient wouldn't wake up for days. We sure learned that pentothal was accumulative.
>
> I didn't do any cases that were in the abdomen, since there was a real anesthetist who could drop ether and had been trained in a real hospital. We were called "Pentothal Pushers."[81]

Draper chose to continue in her anesthesia career. She first applied to Oxford, but her acceptance was canceled when "they found out I was a woman and a nurse, too." She returned to the United States, and enrolled at Barnes Hospital, St. Louis, studying under Helen Lamb.

In spite of the diversity—and sometimes desperate nature—of wartime anesthesia training, the performance record was impressive. As

Baltz reported: "A brilliant testimony of the service record of the Army Medical Department and the Army nurse anesthetist is that approximately 96 per cent of those battle wounded who reached Army hospitals alive were saved, as compared with about 92 per cent in World War I. The nurse anesthetist, whether civilian or Army trained, did a magnificent job in the service."[82]

A "High Type of Service"

As historians of nursing know, retrieving the records of even their most significant contributions is difficult at best, and usually results in a process known as "quilting,"—that is, the gathering of bits and pieces of material to create an evocative collage of the elusive whole. What follows is such a collection of nurse anesthetist contributions to the World War II effort, contributions to both the Atlantic and Pacific war theaters.

In her own presentation to the AANA, Lieutenant Colonel Baltz chose one example of the "high type of service that nurse anesthetists gave despite the fact that military emergencies limited the amount of training that they received":

During the intense-combat period of 1944, a 2,000 bed hospital in Italy was receiving an average of 400 battle casualties daily. Two years before, this hospital unit had gone overseas with four anesthetists. One of these was a registered anesthetist, and the others had received brief training in obstetric anesthesia in civilian institutions. While this unit was in Africa, it became evident that additional nurse anesthetists would be needed when the unit moved closer to the front lines. Consequently, a request was made that members of the general nursing staff volunteer for training in anesthesia. This training was only of three months' duration. At the end of that time, these volunteers were thrown into a situation in which 100 operations were being performed every 24 hours.

In this situation, it was obviously impossible to give a standard course in anesthesia to the nurse anesthetists. There were not enough hours in the day to care for the patients and at the same time provide for formal classroom instruction. However, this particular hospital had an excellent medical anesthetist, and he spent most of his time going from operating room to operating room to supervise these volunteer nurse anesthetists in giving anesthetics. In this hospital, over 5,000 anesthetics were given during a six months' period and not one death or complication occurred as a result of the anesthesia.[83]

In November 1945 the AANA *Bulletin* printed a letter from member Evelyn K. King, a graduate of Charity Hospital School of Anesthesia, New Orleans. In it she described her experiences in England:

England has proven quite interesting. I have been overseas eighteen months. All of this time with the exception of one month has been spent with the same unit. The other month was with the 96th General Hospital which activated in Texas. When we arrived in England it was revealed that the 96th would function as a neuropsychiatric hospital. There was little need for surgeons and anesthetists so as a result, I came to the 232nd Station Hospital as an anesthetist.

We have had some interesting and exciting times in work as well as in play. Our unit at one time was divided—half in Southampton and my half at Tidworth. Tidworth is an Old English Post; incidentally it is where Montgomery trained his 5th Army. I was the only anesthetist there. Spinals which the surgeons gave, gas-oxygen-ether (G.O.E.), and Pentothal were used chiefly there. There have only been two anesthetists with this unit at all times; a medical officer and myself.

Lieutenant Colonel Ralph Tovell from Mayo Brothers is the Chief Consultant in Anesthesia in the European Operating Theater. When we first came over, he held a one-week school for anesthetists. Here we learned the pros and cons of anesthesia in the E.T.O. and Army. The course was an instructive one. We also met many interesting men of anesthesia.

Another interesting experience was a month of detached service with a general hospital which was the chest center of the E.T.O. Here Colonel Tourof from New York was the Chief of the Chest Service.

Major Adelman from Mt. Sinai, New York, was the Chief of Anesthesia. Cyclopropane was used occasionally. It was interesting to note because there are only two or three hospitals over here permitted to use cyclopropane. The cyclopropane is not issued to a unit or hospital, but to an anesthesiologist. Major Adelman happened to be the Junior Consultant in Anesthesia for that medical center. However, G.O.E. was used chiefly in chest cases. The patient was intubated in each instance where the pleura was opened.

Major Adelman taught anesthesia. He gave interesting courses and took great pride in his nurse students as well as the medical ones. He has formerly taught medical students in New York.

King was also able to send along information on two fellow AANA members, both of whom were also Charity Hospital School of Anesthesia graduates: Lieutenant Margaret Moore came to England with King, then went on to India, and Lieutenant Lorine Slagle, who came over with the 96th General Hospital, but had since been transferred to a field evacuation hospital.[84]

Another AANA member, Lieutenant (j.g.) Ruth Toenberg, NC, USNR, received a citation for meritorious service while aboard a hospital ship. In a ceremony on June 20, 1945, at the US Naval Hospital, Seattle (the first such ceremony held at this Hospital to honor a nurse), Commanding Officer Captain F. C. Hill presented Lieutenant Toenberg with the citation that was issued from the Commander of the Service Force, US Pacific Fleet. It read:

> For meritorious service in the line of her profession as a nurse on board a U.S. hospital ship sailing in enemy waters from November, 1943, to April, 1945. Through her able assistance, exceptional ability and tireless devotion to duty the care of the wounded was conducted in an efficient and salutary manner. Her deft, gentle and sympathetic nursing care contributed substantially to the alleviation of the suffering of the wounded and minimized loss of life.
>
> Her personal influence and encouragement have inspired the crippled, maimed and blinded to renew their hope and revitalized their interest in life. The patience and physical endurance displayed by her during long and arduous hours was outstanding. Her exemplary conduct throughout was in keeping with the highest traditions of the Naval Service.

The citation was signed by Vice Admiral W. W. Smith, USN.[85]

Army Nurse Captain Clara A. Vezina, another AANA member, received a citation from the Headquarters, United States Army Forces of the Western Pacific, which read:

> For meritorious achievement in Biak, The Netherland East Indies, from 7 November 1944 to 2 June 1945, in connection with military operations against the enemy. Captain Vezina was chief nurse anesthetist in the surgical service of a large hospital during a period in which it cared for large numbers of medical and surgical casualties evacuated from the Southern Philippines and Luzon campaigns. Under a heavy census of patients which frequently numbered over fifty per cent above rated capacity, she held complete responsibility for the proper administration of anesthesia to all casualties undergoing operative surgery. In addition, she maintained close supervision over other nurse anesthetists on the staff and contributed much extra effort to instruction and training. By her consistently superior performance, initiative, and devotion to duty in the per-

formance of arduous and exacting tasks, Captain Vezina made an important contribution to the proper care of the sick and wounded in the Southwest Pacific Area.[86]

Annie Mealer, an army nurse anesthetist from Walter Reed, had been placed in charge of the Corregidor Hospital, the Philippines, in September, 1941. She had a staff of twelve nurses and about five hundred patients. She was to spend three years as a Japanese prisoner of war. To her friend, Edith Aynes, she later wrote:

After the bombing of Pearl Harbor, on December 9th, we were ordered to set up a hospital section in Malinta Tunnel. Taking Sergeant Clark and a number of medical corpsmen from Topside Hospital, we cleared the tunnel of all unnecessary equipment that had become useless from storage, and scrubbed the place from top to bottom. There were only a couple of water spigots for the entire hospital, and no toilet facilities. The electricians were working on the lights and ventilating system. We transferred our patients from Topside Hospital down the steep drive to the tunnel hospital while the Jap planes flew over us, and the schrapnel from the anti-aircraft guns fell too close to be comfortable. The nurses' uniforms were changed from the crisp white to a khaki skirt and a soldier shirt, two suits per nurse, which was to be their only wardrobe for three years.

Christmas 1941, brought the Higher Commissioner and Mrs. Sayer and son, Janet White and Anibel Newcomb, private secretaries, and other members of the High Commission staff. All had to be stuffed into cramped quarters with insufficient air, light, and water. A clean towel and sheet when it could be spared about every two weeks. They all fell into the hospital routine helping to make surgical dressings and other supplies as efficiently as any surgical nurse. President Quezon, family and physician, nurse and staff all had to be quartered in the hospital section. It was necessary to move the nurses' quarters up to a lateral near the middle of the tunnel. To do this I had to have permission from my commanding officer, so I rode up to Topside Hospital with one of the medical officers to consult him regarding this change. After a short visit with him I walked down the steps to the nurses' quarters one ledge below the hospital. There were some nurses waiting for me who had just been evacuated from Manila. The air raid signal went off and we only had time to jump into a ditch a few feet away from the nurses' quarters. The Jap bombs missed very little on the island that day. It sounded as if the whole world were being blown away. They strafed our quarters and I could hear the bark of a machine gun over us, but not one of us was injured. The medical officer with whom I had ridden up to the hospital that morning was shot through the heart. We were literally snatched from that ditch by Colonel Bowler's driver, and rushed to the tunnel in a car between waves of bombers. In the tunnel I threw my helmet off, tied my hair up in a piece of gauze, and checked the shock wards to see if they had adequate help. Then to the operating room where I gave anesthetics to one casualty after another. When all the casualties had been cleared I realized that we hadn't eaten since morning. It was then 8 p.m. Also, our water supply had been hit in the bombing which caused us to have to ration our water to one drink a day, and two of fruit juice for our patients. Not a drop could be spared for brushing teeth or for washing faces of the feverish patients. The seawater that had been filtered and flavored with coffee made us more thirsty. I dreamed of fresh, cool water running over stones, green grass, and fresh air. After about forty-eight hours, wells were dug and water was available in small quantities.

When there was a lull in the bombing, the nurses were allowed to go over to Bataan on their time off duty. I had the Chinese cook bake the largest chocolate cake that would go in the stove to take to the nurses on Bataan. Also boxes of surgical dressings that were made by the civilian women and badly needed on Bataan. . . .

As the bombing and shelling of Corregidor intensified, we were too busy to leave our duties as the casualties were heavy. Our only recreation was a bridge game in the mess lateral, after 7 p.m. or a venture to the entrance of the tunnel for a breath of air.

The order came to prepare to take care of nurses from Bataan. The beds had to be triple-decked, but where I was to get the linen to cover them I did not know, as the water supply prevented little laundry work. After scouting around I finally managed one sheet per bed. The explosions were so great over in Bataan they shook the tunnel and I didn't think I would get the nurses all in one piece; but about noon, they began to come in one by one, tired and dirty from diving into fox holes. I swallowed the lump in my throat and managed to get enough towels and water to clean them up. Soup was all I had to offer them. Several of them were running temperatures of 102–103 from malaria. In a couple of days Colonel Elms of the Quartermaster department had them all outfitted in coveralls. Nothing was too much trouble for him. He also had a "Magic Lamp."

The shelling and bombing was so constant then, we did not dare go near the entrance. I worked from 12 to 14 hours in the operating room and would go across to the medical supply to listen to a couple of chapters from a book the Colonel was reading aloud. It seemed to take my mind off the misery around me. It was difficult at times to hear his voice above the noise of the shelling.

I was called to the commanding officer's office and told they were evacuating the nurses; a group would leave that night. I was to be ready. I turned and walked out. When I reached the main tunnel, I heard a voice call, "Clear the way for casualties." I looked at the face on the litter as it passed. It was the little G.I. from the Topside switchboard, who had gone to no end of trouble to locate me whenever I was needed. I went back to the operating room to find him badly wounded. As I sat there administering anesthesia to him, I reviewed the cases in the tunnel. They all needed help that only a nurse could give them. I sent word to my commanding officer that I would stay with them. Here in this tunnel choked with shell smoke and misery was a group of people that meant more to me than anything else.

The Physical Therapy Aide, "Bee" [Brunetta Kuelthau], held some coffee while I swallowed it. No time to stop as I went from one case to another. All night the casualties streamed in. The Japs were landing on Corregidor. I looked at my nurses whose faces were pale and tired. They moved quietly, never uttering a word, as the concussion of the shells blew their skirts tight about their legs.

A voice over the radio announced that General Wainwright would surrender—our brave commander who was afraid of nothing, as I have seen him sit and smoke an after-dinner cigar while the Jap shells whistled near by. We worked on, stopping only long enough to catch a couple of hours' sleep, losing track of time— Japanese officers inspecting our equipment, making pictures of us. The nurses falling ill with dysentery; the G.I.'s saying the flies had air superiority; our officers and soldiers streaming in from the camp on the hot sands of the beach where they had been placed by the Japs—they, too, suffering from dysentery, skin infections, and just plain exhaustion.

We were forbidden to speak to our officers, but Colonel Pete sent me a note saying the Japs were taking him to Manila and would I take care of the picture he was sending me of his little boy, the dearest possession he had. He came to Santo Tomas to see me a couple of times after I had been sent over there, and later was killed aboard the Japanese prison ship on December 15, 1944.

I fell ill with dengue fever, and when the Japs took us to Manila aboard a troop ship, I threw my cape down on the deck to lie on it and prayed that the wind would blow the fumes of the stale fish in another direction. I looked around at the nurses in their various uniforms of coveralls and skirts. They had grown slender as reeds, but were smiling over some secret rumor about liberation—not realizing they had nearly three more years of hard work and starvation.

The Jap who inspected my baggage at Santo Tomas came across a picture of Colonel Pete. A broad grin spread across his face showing a row of yellow teeth. "Ah, an American officer. Killed on Bataan?" Ha, ha, ha—his laugh rang out over the squalid scene. I made no reply. He who laughs last, laughs best.

Mealer and her fellow prisoners were released by American troops in February 1945. They were awarded the Philippine Defense Ribbon.[87]

In her informative study, *American Women in the 1940s: The Home Front and Beyond,* Susan M. Hartmann has demonstrated that the gender stereotypes that existed in American society as a whole were, not surprisingly, mirrored in the military. So it was that military public relations efforts and news reports tended to focus on the social clichés: "Newsreels frequently referred to women as 'girls' or 'gals' and stressed the most dramatic as well as the more frivolous aspects of servicewomen's experience, such as their underwear and their patronage of beauty shops."[88] So it was that, even in the face of the heroic contributions by nurse anesthetists, a radio drama such as the following, reported by Aynes, could be presented by a military public relations office:

> Writers in the Bureau of Public Relations preferred to emphasize the woman in the story rather than the Army nurse because of the desire of the WACs to minimize the difference between the work done by the nurses and the work done by WAC medical and surgical technicians. For this reason, nurses were depicted as "morale boosters," "just the touch of a woman's hand," etc.
>
> At one time, the Army Service Forces branch of Public Relations decided to write a series of shows about the Medical Department, one show for each category of personnel: physical therapist, veterinarian, dentist, doctor, and so on through the nine Corps that comprised the professional side of the Medical Department. The captain who worked on the Nurse Corps show was married to a WAC captain. He had chosen an operating-room scene on the battlefield and he described the surgical nurse and the nurse-anesthetist working with the surgeons on a badly wounded soldier. In the course of the story the nurse-anesthetist became emotional over the soldier's condition and began to cry, finally sobbing openly.
>
> When the script was sent to me for technical clearance, I asked the captain for a conference. If we were to have only *one* show, I was hoping nurses could be shown under at least a favorable light. I objected to the sobs as being unprofessional.

"She's a woman, isn't she?" the captain demanded to know. "Are you trying to tell me nurses don't cry?"

"Of course nurses cry," I admitted. "I've even cried myself. But a nurse-anesthetist who could not control her emotions in a busy operating room under fire in France would not *be* there if she could not control them. No surgeon has time for a crying anesthetist."

The captain fingered the script. "The trouble with you is that you don't know anything about radio."

Aynes replied, "The trouble with you is that you don't know anything about nursing."[89] Her protestations notwithstanding, the show was broadcast as written.

The irony of the willingness to exploit a frivolous sexual stereotype is redoubled with the revelation that the life and death symbolism of nurses was not lost on military authorities—and did not go unexploited on the battlefield. Aynes reports that the decision to take nurses to the Anzio Beachhead, where hospitals were "nestled in with combat units," was a deliberate one. The surgeon of the Fifth Army, Brigadier General Joseph I. Martin, in his official report to the Surgeon General, said:

It can now be told that at one time, the removal of all nurses from the beachhead was considered. There were sound reasons to support this proposal. And yet, after a hard-headed estimate of the matter, it was decided that they should remain. Had the nurses been removed, the act would have betrayed to the combat troops the gravity of their own plight.

Nurses certainly *are not* expendable, but in a situation as critical as that which developed on the beachhead—when subjective factors determined whether a line would hold or crack—these nurses assumed a major symbolic importance. It was different on the front before Cassino where space alone made it impossible for combat troops to know what was happening to medical installations in their rear. On the beachhead, any single unit knew everything there was to know about all other units. The presence of the nurses on the beachhead constituted a ringing affirmation of our determination to hold what we had.

No enumeration of the elusive factors which enabled our men to hold their ground at Anzio can overlook the role played by the nurses there. Certainly no combat troops who were at Anzio will fail to honor those heroic women, six of whom lie buried side by side with Infantrymen, tank drivers, artillery men and others in the American cemetery on the beachhead.[90]

AANA's Wartime Pursuit of Educational Goals

At the beginning of this chapter, it was said that the tasks faced by the American Association of Nurse Anesthetists in the 1930s and 1940s were enormous: legal challenges from without, a struggle within to determine a path for achievement of standardization and accreditation of schools, and—as the World War II vignettes above dramatically make clear—extraordinary complications for its educational plans stemming from the necessity of emergency-trained nurse anesthetists. But, because the Association leadership clearly recognized the threat of irregular training to its own educational goals, it doggedly pursued them even while bearing the grueling work loads caused by the war, with its shortage of nurse anesthetists in both the military and civilian arenas.

In May 1942 the Association published an eight-page recruiting brochure (anonymously authored by Gertrude Fife), titled, "Anesthesia: A Career for the Graduate Nurse." In it she presented the Association's position in the face of the wartime emergency:

The need for nurse anesthetists both in civilian and Army hospitals is becoming increasingly urgent. In order to meet the situation, many Schools of Anesthesia have increased the student body. The degree of expansion is limited, however, because in order to qualify for membership in the American Association of Nurse Anesthetists, each anesthetist must have administered a certain number of anesthetics during her training. The American Association has been opposed to lowering the standards by allowing the student to be graduated with less clinical experience than necessary to prepare her properly for work in active surgical clinics. The Association has therefore encouraged the establishment of schools in hospitals equipped to offer training in this field.[91]

Fife's brochure, which included a history of nurse anesthesia and of the national Association, as well as its "Educational Program," along with the "Organization Plan *Recommended* for Schools of Anesthesia" (emphasis added) and "Requirements for Admission to Schools of Anesthesia," was a considerable success. In November 1942 the *Bulletin of the American Association of Nurse Anesthetists* reported: "This booklet has had wonderful acceptance. Doctors who are heads of allied associations and hospital journals have been most complimentary. The American Journal of Nursing asked to report parts of this brochure in their Journal. The Science Research Institute of Chicago, publishers of vocational material, are reprinting it." Furthermore, "As a good-will measure, and in the interests of public education, hundreds of these pamphlets have gone out from Headquarters to schools of anesthesia, schools of nursing, hospital superintendents, school editors of many newspapers, and to medical libraries."[92]

In the same year, a Special Committee was established by the association to organize the mechanics for the certification of nurse anesthetists. Committee members were Miriam Shupp (Chair), Gertrude Fife, and Helen Lamb. The following "Resolution" was adopted unanimously and published in the November 1942 *Bulletin:*

Whereas: The increased need for anesthetists in the armed forces has created an acute shortage of nurse anesthetists, and

Whereas: It is the earnest desire of the Board of Trustees of the American Association of Nurse Anesthetists not only to maintain the standards already attained, but to raise the standards during this period, and

Whereas: There are now various hospitals opening schools of anesthesia, offering courses of at least six months' duration, but whose graduates are from time to time making application for membership in this Association,

Therefore Be It Resolved:

1. That during this period the standards of this Association shall not only be maintained, but shall be raised, by inaugurating a program of certification by examination and certification by waiver, thus requiring that the membership in its entirety shall be a certified membership;
2. That each individual applying for membership, in order to become certified, shall have the qualifications now required by this Association and shall be required to take, in addition, an examination conducted by this Association.
3. That all nurse anesthetists already members of this Association and eligible to become certified, shall become certified by waiver in lieu of examination during a designated period, or forfeit the right to membership.
4. That the sum of $10.00, apart from the annual dues, be set as the certification fee, such monies to be used to meet the expenses of the program and to further advance the educational program.
5. That this resolution shall be printed in the convention proceedings, and that proper and sufficient advance notice of the inauguration of the program of certification by examination and certification by waiver, shall appear in the official organ of this Association, the Bulletin of the American Association of Nurse Anesthetists.[93]

In November 1943 President Rosalie McDonald reported that AANA membership growth in the past year had been 413, "exceed[ing] those received last year by 100, and only a rigid adherence to the policy of requiring high standards for membership prevented a phenomenal increase." Moreover, "A number of Schools of Anesthesia are being opened in an effort to meet the demand for a greater number of active anesthetists. That these new schools are eager to cooperate in meeting the educational requirements of the Association is evidenced by the many requests from hospitals for the recommended curriculum. These schools are anxious to graduate students who are eligible for membership in our organization and they have been given direction and assistance by Miss Helen Lamb, Chairman of the Committee on Education."[94]

In response to still-increasing demands, the Committee on Education (Helen Lamb, Chair, Janet McMahon, and Miriam Shupp) announced in November 1944 that it had prepared a bulletin, "Essentials of an Accepted School of Anesthesia for Graduate Nurses." Its stated purpose was to "aid adequately staffed institutions to increase facilities for such proper training, but vigorously deprecate any even temporary debasement of the high standards of education that must of necessity exist in, and are vital to, acceptable preparation for entrance to our field."[95]

Thus, the fact that great numbers of individuals and institutions looked to the national Association for direction and guidance in establishing programs testified to the fact that the Association was coming, in fact, to be viewed as an accrediting agency—years before it legally became one.

Although the Association was one of the few domestic organizations allowed to continue its meetings during the war, activities necessarily slowed as the war dragged on. For example, in November 1942 President Helen Lamb was able to report that, "during this period almost 25 percent of all the schools of anesthesia for nurse anesthetists that have functioned for a year or more, have been surveyed by our field visitors."[96] But, in May 1944 Executive Secretary Anne M. Campbell had to report that the school survey had been "temporarily suspended due to the war." But, she continued, "the results of the examination should provide a basis for judging the thoroughness of the schools."[97]

Early optimism regarding the war effort was gradually eroded. As early as October 1942 President Helen Lamb could already discuss potential postwar problems of the Association, and, one year later, President Rosalie McDonald could say that, "Throughout the world, a feeling of optimism is becoming increasingly evident. We cannot yet foresee what the future holds, but at least we hope that soon we shall face the problems of peace rather than those of war."[98] But, due to ill health, McDonald had to resign in 1944, bringing Hazel Blanchard into office. The contents of the *Bulletin of the American Association of Nurse Anesthetists* steadily diminished, reflecting the lack of time for study and resources for scientific and academic research during the war years.

In December 1944 Agatha Hodgins, writing from Chatham, Massachusetts, could only offer words of encouragement to persevere, with good cheer, in the face of destruction. Taking as her text, Shelley's lines, "Many a green isle needs must be / In the deep wide sea of Misery," she wrote:

> Never in the history of mankind has necessity been more pressing in its need, or duty more imperative in its call to create, within this present chaos of destruction, citadels of good will from which to combat the forces of evil rampant in the world.
>
> It is therefore of immense importance that all organizations designed to dispense and perpetuate good to humanity will be, during these hazardous times, nourished, strengthened and made more vitally useful, through the spirit and endeavors of their membership. This responsibility calls, even in times of great personal stress and strain, for greater effort, increased devotion, and clear thinking on the part of each individual member. It calls upon all for constant resistance to a pressing sense of futility and discouragement, which present catastrophic events impose. It calls for the exercise, often under harassing circumstances, of courage, fortitude and hopeful good cheer—in a good cause. It calls for the cultivation of common sense—the exercise of proportionate discrimination in the choice of real values, in determining a course of action most sure to serve best the common cause. It calls for restraint in not judging too hastily the force and significance of rapidly changing circumstances—being neither overly optimistic about gains or too pessimistic over losses. Imperatively it calls for faith—an abiding faith in the ultimate triumph of righteousness over the forces of evil. To be productive, such faith must be implemented into constructive service; to be effectual it must be constantly reinforced by resolution to do our part, however small, in efforts to end this terrible and devastating war.
>
> Those entrusted with the guidance of such associations—forced to meet and overcome unparalled circumstances which threaten to nullify past achievements and jeopardize present progress—may be fortified by the knowledge that agencies for good have in the past stamped out, in some cases, and greatly ameliorated, in others, conditions which, throughout the ages, threatened the freedom

and welfare of mankind and impeded the progress of civilization. Confidently then we hold firm to the belief that through coordinated, well-directed efforts and good will—present chaos will be reduced to order, intolerable conditions overcome, and this good earth become a place where all peoples may work together in freedom for the common good. The immense and vital part all branches of medical service will play in this continuing task can—because of its greatness—be now only dimly conceived. They will in very truth be "green island" in "the wide deep sea of misery" now encompassing the earth. . . .

In a wider sense our endeavors will take on the garment of permanency *if* we regard our Association as a medium through which may be brought into being "flowering islands" of fruitful service to enrich the life of our nation. And let us all daily pray that such "green islands" may increase in number until the world's "wide deep sea of misery" becomes a green productive land, whereon free peoples may work together in creative efforts to cultivate and perpetuate for all time the arts and sciences of peace—the only sure wall of defense against aggressive forces of evil.[99]

These were to be her last words to the Association. She died suddenly on March 24, 1945. The war years also saw the loss, in 1943, of her mentor, Dr. George Washington Crile.[100]

Sadly, Hodgins never lived to see the first Qualifying Examination for membership in the American Association of Nurse Anesthetists, held on June 4, 1945. Ninety-two candidates participated in thirty-nine hospitals in twenty-eight states, and one in Hawaii. Nor did she see the first Institute for Instructors of Anesthesiology, held in Chicago, the week of October 8, 1945. One hundred and thirty-seven nurse anesthetists participated, representing thirty-four states, Hawaii, and four army nurses (the latter anticipating becoming teachers upon return to civilian life). The perseverance and determination of Association leaders during the difficult wartime years quickly came to fruition in peacetime.

· 6 ·

Everything Is Under Control

When the war came to an end, we all hoped that many of our problems would quickly disappear. The end of the war has brought forth not only a hangover of many of our old problems, but many new ones.

Thus AANA President Lucy Richards plaintively reflected in 1947.[1]

One immediate problem for the Association, resulting from its own expansion, occurred in its Executive Office. The Association headquarters had been moved from Cleveland to Chicago in 1937. Only the treasury remained behind. Nine years later, that office was also relocated (though Gertrude Fife, in Cleveland, held the position of treasurer until 1950). The added burden of business proved to be one task too many for the incumbent lay executive secretary: membership dues checks went uncashed, membership cards unsent, letters unanswered.[2]

In February 1948 President Richards announced: "With the growth of the Association, it has been evident that a pressing need for a more efficient co-ordination of activities demanded a change in the method of handling Association affairs in the Executive Office, and an Executive Director with the professional background of an anesthetist."[3] The choice was Florence A. McQuillen, her term of office to begin March 1, 1948. McQuillen had been a staff anesthetist and instructor of anesthesia at the Mayo Clinic. She came there in 1927, at the invitation of Dr. John S. Lundy, head of its Anesthesia Department. Richards's expressed belief that "Miss McQuillen will be able to give more efficient attention to both state and national affairs than has hitherto been possible"[4] was not unrewarded. No single Association leader before or after McQuillen would exercise comparable control over all facets of its business.

A brilliant and powerful personality, McQuillen had the qualities necessary to see the Association through the severe challenges that came after World War II. By 1970, however, those same qualities (her style of leadership perhaps best described as one of "benevolent dictatorship") had lost their appropriateness: the health-care scene had changed dramatically during her twenty-two-year tenure as executive director. But, like Agatha Hodgins, "Mac" would not take "forced" retirement gracefully.

An "Old Problem" Reappears

Anesthesia as a medical specialty was given great impetus from World War II. It resulted not only from the increased complexity of anesthetics, but also from a military structure that encouraged medical specialization and a GI Bill that supported medical residencies. With this newly strengthened position, some of the anesthesiologists (as physician-anesthetists now called themselves) launched a vigorous national public-relations campaign that was pro-anesthesiologist and anti-nurse anesthetist. Their message to the country was that anesthesia was safe only when delivered by a physician.

The major articles in this campaign included "Safer Surgery for 1947," a *Look* magazine photo-essay of January 7, 1947, signed by Lawrence Drake. According to *Hospital Management*, Drake was said to have been hired as a press agent by certain physician anesthesiologists.[5] This particular piece declared: "Bad anesthesia causes more operating-room deaths than surgery. Now many hospitals have physician-anesthetists to protect you." Another Drake essay, "Will You Live Through Your Operation?" appeared in the February, 1947, issue of *Reader's Scope*. Here Drake announced: "Your chances of dying on the operating table are 27 times greater in a poor hospital, and eight times greater in an average hospital, than they are in a good one." He continued: "What makes the radical difference between the good and the bad in our hospitals? It isn't the surgeon." No, it's that, as "the result of the greatest consideration for the patient's safety in the operating room," there exists in "most of our first-class hospitals" "the practice of using only physician-anesthesiologists." Drake's tract built to a concluding image of carnage:

> But how many patients get this care—which every patient deserves. The grim fact is that no more than about five to ten per cent of our hospitals are serviced by P-As [physician-anesthesiologists].

To close this chasm as rapidly as possible the public will have to make its demand felt for more and larger anesthesiology departments in our medical schools. It will have to demand that thousands of residencies in anesthesiology be created in our hospitals. Until the operating rooms of our hospitals are brought into line with the clear requirements of modern anesthesiology, hundreds of Americans will continue to die needlessly on operating tables, sacrificed to ignorance and incompetence.

"Unknown Men in White," a photo-essay in *This Week* magazine of November 23, 1947, by James R. Miller, focused on the work of Drs. Emery A. Rovenstine and Emmanuel M. Papper at Bellevue Hospital. Miller opened with the following scene: "Suppose you're on your way to the operating room. Within a few minutes your life will be in the hands of two people. One is your surgeon. The chances are he knows his business. The other is your anesthetist. Unluckily for you, most anesthetists today are not qualified for their job." Specifically, "a competent anesthetist must have long training and profound medical judgment. The nurses and technicians who give most anesthesia today have neither. This means that most operations today are not as safe as they could be."

The alarming nature of this series of publications, which *Hospital Management* called "barely short of libelous,"[6] caused the Board of Regents of the American College of Surgeons to adopt the following resolution on February 22, 1948:

> The American College of Surgeons regards with deep concern the actions of some physician anesthesiologists in giving the impression to the laity in the public press that it is unsafe for experienced nurse anesthetists to conduct surgical anesthesia. While it supports the increasing tendency of having physician anesthesiologists in charge of surgical anesthesia, it deplores at this time any propaganda for the elimination of the trained nurse anesthetist.
>
> On the contrary, the American College of Surgeons is of the opinion that, in view of the inadequacy in number of physician anesthesiologists and in view of the splendid record of achievement of the nurse anesthetists, institutions engaged in the training of nurses for this purpose should be encouraged to continue their programs.[7]

Two months earlier, the Southern Surgical Association had passed unanimously a similar resolution. This statement made more graphic the dangerous impact of the propaganda tactics:

Although the Southern Surgical Association has been and always will be extremely interested in the advancement of all medical sciences, and particularly in anesthesia because of complete dependence on safe anesthesia for the safe performance of a surgical procedure, it, the Southern Surgical Association, heartily disapproves of the publicity given by certain newspapers and popular lay magazines to the statements sponsored by a group of anesthesiologists who are seeking to discredit the well trained nurse anesthetist and to compel surgeons to operate only if anesthetics are administered by physician anesthetists.

This attempt to persuade the public that there is grave danger in a surgical operation if the anesthetist is not a certified medical specialist is already decreasing the number of efficient well-trained nurse anesthetists and forcing surgeons to perform recently developed complicated operations with anesthetics administered by young hospital interns or general practitioners, neither of whom have special training or experience in the administration of an anesthetic.[8]

Thus, the danger was that there would be a return to the very conditions of practice that made necessary the presence of the nurse anesthetist in the field.

Even the American Medical Association Board of Trustees, in response to a request from the AANA, "voted to condemn publicity that is not based on a scientific understanding and that does not accurately reflect the prevailing situation."[9]

It seems especially ironic that this energetic anti-nurse anesthetist attack occurred at a time of a general shortage of all trained anesthetists. Miriam Shupp of Lakeside Hospital, Cleveland, described the need for nurse anesthetists: "Letters, telegrams, and long distance calls come in almost daily to our department office requesting nurse anesthetists—requests that we cannot fill. This same situation exists in other hospitals conducting training programs in anesthesia for nurses, and I understand, many requests are also received at the Association Executive Office." These requests, "some of them urgent pleas," came from the Veterans Administration; from hospitals faced with increased patient care (some hospitals expanding existing nurse anesthetist service, other hospitals initiating it); from dentists, surgeons, industry, and the military. Shupp, therefore, called for an expansion of Association efforts in encouraging the training of a greater number of "well qualified" nurse anesthetists.[10]

The viewpoint of a hospital Director was presented by Dr. Kenneth B. Babcock in a 1949 paper, "The Hospital's Dilemma": "There are 6,400 general hospitals in the United States, embracing 1,400,000 beds. There are about 4,500 registered nurse anesthetists and 400 registered [Board certified] physician anesthetists, plus 1,000 unregistered physician anesthetists. That means about one anesthetist per hospital." Since at Babcock's hospital alone, there were over 18,000 anesthetics administered per year, "obviously, there is a very great shortage."[11] (Interestingly, one solution to the shortage proffered by Babcock was that nurse anesthetists train their own "practical anesthetists," assistants who could "handle normal cases, give routine anesthetics, and know enough to call for your help when needed." Unlike the AANA nurse anesthetist, the "practical anesthetist" would not have to "spend hours on a curriculum of history of anesthesia, physiology and pharmacology of anesthetic agents, and a host of other academic considerations.")[12]

One reason for the anti-nurse anesthetist publicity campaign was indicated in the "Unknown Men in White" article. There, Rovenstine stated that one "immediate" postwar goal of anesthesiologists was "to have at least one thoroughly qualified anesthetist [physician specialist] in every hospital. He should be available—not downstairs drinking coffee—to handle any kind of emergency and to supervise the nurses and technicians who will be doing most of the work for a long time to come." But another goal at this time was to change the structure of third-party insurance payments. In 1938, anesthesiologists succeeded in obtaining hospital payment by fee rather than salary, while nurse anesthetists continued to be salaried hospital employees. The new voluntary hospital insurance plans *had* included anesthesia as an auxiliary *hospital* service. Anesthesiologists wanted to be recognized as providing a *medical* service, thus having access to direct third-party reimbursement, a source of professional autonomy and significantly increased income. In the course of reaching this goal, public protests over the resultant increased anesthesia costs—e.g., headlines such as "Anesthesia Costs Rise as Doctors Take Over"[13]—had to be overcome. The portrayal of anesthesia as a deadly risk unless conducted by a physician could only help to justify the added cost.

As for the AANA response to the hostile public relations campaign, Gertrude Fife declared:

What is to be our answer to this unfortunate publicity? We do not wish to behave like the ostrich, nor do we wish to engage in fruitless rebuttal. The publication of such articles should certainly be discouraged. However, the positive answer to the challenge is to continue to improve the standards of the nurse anesthetist and to give the medical profession the same loyal service that has been given in the past, in order that the nurse anesthetist may receive the recognition she deserves.

Fife concluded with a homey adage that communicated her unshakable confidence in the nurse anesthetist: "For those who would challenge the position of the nurse anesthetist, there is an old saying that should someone 'build a better mousetrap, the world will clear a path to his door.'"[14]

This is not to suggest that there were not those within the Association who wanted to "retaliate with an intensive publicity campaign," as well as others who urged "inaction." But, as President Lucy Richards reported, the Board of Trustees decided on a "middle course." By allowing other professional associations, prominent medical figures, and hospital-related publications to affirm the record of nurse anesthetists, "our tormenters have been chastized by their peers, and we have maintained our professional integrity."[15]

The 1947 "Anti-Adriani Bylaw"

In 1941, Dr. John Adriani left Bellevue Hospital in New York and his mentor, Dr. Emery Rovenstine, to assume the directorship of the Anesthesia Department at Charity Hospital, New Orleans. At the time, Charity Hospital was one of the largest hospitals in the world. Serving indigent patients, it had a total of 3,550 beds and a housestaff of 450 interns and residents. With a staff of forty nurses, Adriani had to cover more than forty anesthetizing areas.

There had been some concern at Charity that Adriani would abolish its School of Anesthesia for Nurses, replacing it with a medical residency program. But the demands of patient care left him with no choice but to employ nurses. Committed to giving all of his anesthesia students the best training possible, he strengthened both the didactic and clinical programs. He also doubled the enrollment. Thus, Adriani was a highly visible anesthesiologist directing a major school of nurse anesthesia.

In 1947, in another postwar anti-nurse anesthetist action, the Board of Directors of the American Society of Anesthesiologists "adopted a statement in its bylaws to the effect that it was unethical for an anesthesiologist to participate in the training of nurses"; it also "precluded giving lectures at the annual meetings for the American Association of Nurse Anesthetists."[16] In addition, Adriani was personally informed by Dr. Paul Wood, secretary of the American Board of Anesthesiology, that the board was "seriously considering" the revocation of certification of any anesthesiologist who trained nurse anesthetists.

Ever a man to speak his mind, Adriani later recalled that he told Wood that "his responsibility and loyalty were to patient care and not to any concept or philosophy that anesthesiologists, the ASA or ABA might have," and that "if nurses were to be relied upon to render patient care, they should be taught as much as possible so that patients received the best they were capable of giving."[17] Promising to respond with a federal lawsuit to any revocation of his certification, Adriani heard no more and continued his work. The so-called "anti-Adriani bylaw," however, was not rescinded until 1964.[18] The impact of this ASA/ABA pressure on other anesthesiologists cannot be assessed.

AANA Accreditation Goal Achieved

In the midst of this controversy, Gertrude Fife had reminded the Association that the best response to criticism was "to continue to improve the standards of the nurse anesthetist." It will be recalled that it was Fife (following Karsner) who, at the first national convention in 1933, called for the creation of a list of "accredited" schools in order to assure employers of a nurse anesthetist's qualifications. The war brought a temporary halt to the program in 1944, but the serious postwar problems made it imperative to resume the work.

The American Hospital Association Council on Professional Practice also recognized the need, and in 1945 encouraged the AANA to take definite steps to put the plan into effect. In May 1946 a Joint Committee of the AHA and the AANA was held in Cleveland, with Dr. Frank Bradley of Barnes Hospital presiding. One result was the creation of two AANA standing committees: an Approval Committee and an Advisory to the Approval Committee. Although it was agreed at the AHA/AANA meeting that the AANA would be the accrediting body, the Advisory to the Approval Committee (Helen Lamb, Chair) worked closely with the AHA Council on Professional Practice.

Progress was still slow. In 1948, the new executive director, Florence McQuillen, familiarizing herself with the situation, declared, "It was tragic to me to find that the entire work, long hard hours of work with one of the Committees this year, [duplicated] the same work that had been done as long as seven years ago. There has been no continuity of committee activity. That, I think, is tragic, and I do think we can remedy it, I hope."[19]

Finally, with a renewed pledge of support from the AHA Council on Professional Practice, the plan for the accreditation of schools of anesthesia for nurses was unanimously approved at the Association's annual meeting in September 1950. Also accepted was an increase in membership dues to finance the accreditation program. An important point was made by Dr. Charles T. Dolezal, assistant director of the American Hospital Association: "Nurse anesthetists, like other professional groups, should not only improve their service to the public, but also set standards for practice."[20] Though three advisors were appointed to the accreditation program (originally Dr. Eugene S. Lawler, Dr. Raymond N. Lowe, and Dr. Adam R. Gilliland, all faculty members of Northwestern University's Department of Education),[21] it was the practicing nurse anesthetists themselves who shaped it, a significant act of professional autonomy:

> Those who know the most about the work—the anesthetists themselves—are to formulate the criteria for accreditation through the medium of workshops conducted by the accrediting advisors. This is at once an honored and weighty responsibility to which every best effort will be brought. In setting the accreditation program into motion those concerned have a wealth of experience from which to draw—experience gained from the Association's other educational programs.[22]

The AANA accreditation program for schools of anesthesia for nurses went into effect on January 19, 1952. Schools established after that date had to meet the criteria at the time of application. Schools already in existence had until December 31, 1953, to meet the standards for full approval. Only graduates of accredited schools would be eligible to take the qualifying examination for membership in the AANA. In February 1954 the Association published a list of seventy-two schools having full approval; thirty-two hospitals with new schools of nurse anesthesia received one-year tentative approval pending investigation. To keep this program vital, in 1960 the Association adopted new minimum requirements for approved schools, as well as a policy of reviewing/revising criteria in ten-year intervals.

In 1956, on the occasion of the twenty-fifth anniversary of the national Association, Gertrude Fife reflected on the significance of such achievements as the accreditation program:

> We are justly proud of our achievements and particularly so when we realize that the work was done by our members. We did not seek grants or solicit large contributions. We started with only a few dollars in the treasury. Women holding full-time, responsible jobs in anesthesia travelled miles over week ends to meet with other members to map out programs. We were fortunate that we had far-seeing men in the hospital and surgical groups interested in our work and our progress. They gave us moral support, advice and the stimulus to go forward. We are grateful to them.[23]

Korea and the HEW Recognition of AANA

In April 1951 Association President Verna Bean published an "Open Letter to the Membership," communicating another call to service of country in the face of the Korean conflict:

> Some of you know that the Office of the Surgeon General has asked that we of the AANA take over the problem of recruitment of nurse anesthetists as well as a long range program for getting more nurses into the field, not only for military but for civilian needs. . . . There is no formal declaration of war, and there is no draft. This means that the only manner by which a service can get personnel is through an appeal to the nurse's sense of moral and patriotic obligation, plus her general desire to tend the wounded. . . . Knowing so many of you personally, I am aware that you have never sacrificed duty or obligation to self. It is only another demand made to us to whom demands are a daily expectation. . . . Officially, all of this is merely an "incident." Nevertheless, in this incident thousands of men are being wounded. . . . Be it war or "incident," the soldier is just as wounded and just as dead. Whatever our belief as to the necessity for this strife, only one fact need concern us: the necessity to care for our men. This is real, and it is here.[24]

It was timely that Bean was in office to issue the appeal. She had served as a nurse anesthetist in World War II, and could speak of the value of that experience.[25]

It was AANA member Lieutenant Mildred L. Rush of Pembroke, New Hampshire, who was named the 1953 "Woman of the Year" by the Women's National Press Club. Selected to represent all nurses serving in Korea, she was chosen because of her outstanding record during fifteen months' service there:

> Nurses serving with mobile Army surgical hospitals are volunteers, serving units moving close to the front lines which perform operations on men too seriously wounded to risk transfer back to a field or base hospital. At the end of six months of such duty, nurses may be transferred to safer zones. Lieutenant Rush, however, volunteered for additional duty at the front lines.[26]

Captain Mary "Mollie" M. Younger was another nurse anesthetist honored for her work in Korea. She was selected to be part of an army group discussing the Korean experience in a television program, "The Big Story," produced by the Army Signal Corps. Younger's own story was published in the *AANA News Bulletin,* and is of special interest because of the scarcity of commentary on this period:

> I arrived in Korea August 4, 1950 and was assigned to the 8076 Mobile Army Surgical Hospital . . . which was attached to various divisions at different times. Our first set up was in a cotton mill. Amazing, but true . . . the Korean people operating this mill did not seem a bit disturbed and kept right on spinning their cotton and making winter uniforms for their Army.
>
> The Mobile Army Surgical Hospital has excellent equipment and highly trained personnel capable of caring for any surgical emergency. The staff includes 14 doctors, of whom six are surgeons, one internist, one radiologist, four general duty medical officers, two anesthetists, twelve Army Corps officers, two Medical Service Corps officers, warrant officer and ninety enlisted men. For an ordinary 60-bed hospital, at first glance it would appear that this unit is most generously supplied with professional talent. The reason for this is that each patient admitted is critically wounded, and requires extensive resuscitative and supportive care before and after operation. He ordinarily requires large quantities of blood, oxygen, and continuous suction, in addition to skilled professional care. He is the type of patient who requires round-the-clock nursing and constant attention.
>
> When set up in a factory or mill, a warehouse was used. If in a school building the auditorium was used or if under canvas at least an 8 sectional tent was set aside for this purpose. Our first set-up was in a cotton mill. We made space available in one section of the mill for our operating room which consisted of 6 improvised tables; 2 portable anesthesia machines; 3 portable suction machines and 4 nasal oxygen units. We prepared our Sodium Pentothal, 2½%, in 1000 cc bottles of normal saline or distilled water. We rigged up several round pans about 40 inches in circumference and 4 inches deep . . . partitioned with bass wood to separate the needles, syringes and the pentothal tubing.
>
> Due to the fact that most of the patients were in shock and a poor risk, we also prepared one bottle of 1½% Sodium Pentothal. We soon discovered that the Koreans, who were so debilitated, weak and in shock required very little anesthesia and on many occasions were able to do endotracheals with about 10 cc of 1½% Sodium Pentothal. We were well supplied with D-Tubo-curare and used only very small doses per case:—20–40 Units the most for one case. . . .
>
> In the early days of the Korean conflict, it was not uncommon to admit over 125–200 casualties daily, with peaks of over 400. To

meet the demands imposed by the heavy casualty load, the hospital was set on an assembly line basis.

The casualty was seen here by a qualified surgeon who carefully evaluated the patient. With supplemental diagnostic aids, he confirmed the diagnosis and decided when the patient was ready for surgery; the priority for him to enter surgery; or the need for continued resuscitative and supportive measures. Patients were then taken to surgery in the priority designated, and upon completion of the procedure, were sent to the post-operative ward. When parenteral fluids were no longer necessary, suction tubes removed, and the patient was eating, he was then transferred to the holding section to await evacuation. The modes of transportation, depending upon location, consisted of rail, rail-bus, ambulance, train (formerly known as hospital train) or air.

The surgery section during these heavy influxes would operate 2 major abdominal or chest tables, 1 major orthopedic table and 3 minor tables. By doing endotracheals on all major cases we were able to handle two to three cases at one time. . . .

I like to give credit where credit is due . . . to our first-aid men in the front lines who administered prompt and excellent first-aid at the moment of injury. They made it possible for us to save so many more lives.[27]

Returning veterans faced a problem obtaining GI benefits for training in school of nurse anesthesia, since each state had its own Veterans Administration policy concerning so-called "accredited" schools. The Association therefore appealed to the HEW Department for recognition as the proper agency for accrediting these schools, thus allowing veterans to qualify for their benefits. The appeal was successful, and on November 20, 1955, over the signature of Commissioner Brownell of the Department of Health, Education and Welfare, the AANA was notified that it would be so recognized.

Also in 1955, the AANA conducted a national survey of anesthesia services. Questionnaires were sent to all hospital administrators in the United States and its territories and possessions, asking, in part, for the following information: "During the month of January 1955 what persons were giving anesthesia in your hospital; the name and title (R.N., M.D., etc.)." In the replies, nurses were identified variously by the titles "RN," "RNA" (registered nurse anesthetist, used by many non-Association members), and "MAANA" (member, American Association of Nurse Anesthetists). It was clear, therefore, that some title was needed to signify to employers and the public that an individual nurse anesthetist had met the standards required for Association membership. "Certified Registered Nurse Anesthetist" (CRNA) was the choice, and its use became effective in 1957.

Affirming the "Nurse" in Nurse Anesthetist

Perhaps the greatest irony in the history of American anesthesia professions is that *both* nurse and physician practitioners had to struggle—sometimes with others, sometimes with themselves—to find an identity within the health-care structure. Physicians fought to gain acceptance by their colleagues, to win recognition that theirs was a legitimate medical specialty. Nurses struggled with self-definition before accepting themselves as a clinical specialty within nursing. Agatha Hodgins's own anger with nursing for not responding to her vision left the nurse anesthetists a legacy of alienation from the larger group. It was somewhat portentous, then, that the May 1946 issue of the *Journal of the American Association of Nurse Anesthetists*, which contained a lengthy obituary for Hodgins, also published a panel discussion titled, "The Nurse Anesthetist's Plans for Tomorrow's Responsibilities." The latter contained observations from a director of nursing education that did, indeed, signal the future relationship of nurse anesthetists with nursing.

Madeline McConnell first reminded her nurse anesthetist audience that "it is nursing's educational requirements [which] form the basis of your professional standing." She then affirmed: "The American Nurses' Association is interested in the nurse anesthetists as a field of specialization. We watch with interest and with a certain amount of pride your development. We wish you great success and we feel, too, that the Nurses' Association, per se, has a responsibility to see that applicants come to you soundly prepared and, likewise, we are interested in the sound development of the field."[28] These are words Hodgins had wanted to hear in 1909. Nursing was catching up with its first clinical specialty.

The rapprochement took more time. All of nursing was going through a reorganization. The Committee on the Structure of National Nursing Organizations began a study in 1939, with a goal of consolidating the three major national organizations: the National League of Nursing Education, the National Organization for Public Health Nursing, and the American Nurses' Association. Interrupted by World War II, the work resumed in 1944. Three additional groups were then invited to join in the study—the National Association of Colored Graduate Nurses, the Associated Collegiate Schools of Nursing, and the American Association of Industrial Nurses—in the hope that nursing could "solve its own structural problem early enough to preclude its being taken over by unions, the medical profession, or other willing, but uninformed, groups."[29]

In a 1947 address to the AANA, "Strength Through Co-operation," Louise Knapp, Director of Nursing at Washington University, St. Louis, stressed that any resultant new organization of nurses "must make provisions for special interests—surgery, pediatrics, public health, industrial nursing, and anesthesia."[30] In the postwar confusion, the prospect of affiliation with a larger group did appeal to some AANA members. Thus, in 1951, Verna Rice, a charter association member, felt it necessary to refresh memories on the matter of Hodgins's 1932 request for affiliation with the American Nurses' Association. In an "Opinion Review" in the *Journal of the American Association of Nurse Anesthetists,* Rice reprinted the Hodgins/ANA correspondence. Declaring, "we cannot serve two masters at one and the same time," she concluded:

> In view of the foregoing facts, the matter of affiliation was definitely settled some twenty years ago by the American Nurses' Association. There is nothing in common between the two groups; therefore any further consideration concerning this would be disastrous to the well being of the American Association of Nurse Anesthetists, as the end result would be doom by domination, with loss of individuality of our very fine organization.
>
> The American Hospital Association came to our rescue just after the above incident. . . . [It] has been most helpful to our Association in many ways throughout the years and is right at this time working diligently on the accreditation program for schools of anesthesia, which when completed will be of marked value to all concerned. The American Hospital Association is more concerned with the welfare of the nurse anesthetists, as has been evidenced through the years of their co-operation, than could be hoped for from the American Nurses' Association. . . . Why even consider a change when there is nothing to gain.[31]

Another AANA member, Louise Schwarting, in the same issue pointed out that "from the practical standpoint the A.H.A. is perhaps in a better position to understand our problems. In the vast majority of instances the department of anesthesia functions directly under the chief surgeon or the director of the hospital rather than under the director of nurses. . . . Situated as we are, we are free to develop our program to the best of our ability and are helped to do so by both surgeons and hospital administrators . . . Basically we are nurses, and we are in complete sympathy with all efforts being made to improve the education of nurses, but our specialty must always maintain its separate schools for postgraduate study for reasons so obvious that they need not be enumerated."[32] These arguments notwithstanding, at least one AANA state affiliate (Kansas) wrote to the executive director expressing an interest in becoming a section of the ANA.[33] No such formal alliance occurred.

The announcement in the *Journal of the American Association of Nurse Anesthetists* of the actions of the 1952 Biennial Nursing Convention suggested that, in the view of the Association, the reservations expressed by members Rice and Schwarting were justified. The restructuring of nursing organizations produced not one, but two new entities: a revamped American Nurses' Association, whose purpose was the fostering of high standards of nurse practice and the promoting of the general welfare of nurses, and the National League for Nursing (built on the retained charter of the National League for Nursing Education), whose purpose was the fostering of the development and improvement of nursing services and education. The *Journal* notice pointed out that, of all participating associations, the American Association of Industrial Nurses was the "outstanding exception" in its refusal "to lose its autonomy by dissolving to amalgate with the new National League for Nursing." In addition, in the new plan, there was a "lack of provision for the numerous clinical nursing specialties—presumably, according to a comment of the Chair, because representation on the Board of Directors of clinical sections would mean narrow rather than organizational representation."[34] A protest by psychiatric nurses was unsuccessful.

Thus, nurse anesthetists faced what Rice called "doom by domination" from both nursing *and* medicine. They could only continue on a rather solitary path.

Nursing leader Janet Geister (who, it will be recalled, was executive director of the American Nurses' Association in 1932, when Hodgins made her unsuccessful request for affiliation) reflected on the major failure of nursing's reorganization effort in a 1958 address to the AANA. "We must walk together," Geister said, but the 1952 plan "did not recognize the rise of specialist groups, a substantial part of the nursing force, whose internal affairs demand a larger degree of self-government than can be provided within a parent association." She called for unity,

> the kind of unity in which the specialist groups can participate freely, yet retain control over internal affairs. It's the kind of unity that can consolidate for the common good the competence, judgment and good will within nursing. It can be achieved without costly, wearying discussions of framework and bylaws. Its cost is not

in dollars, but in new thinking—and if we will, we can have it tomorrow.[35]

The kind of organization Geister envisioned did not come "tomorrow," but in 1973, with the formation of what came to be called the "National Federation for Specialty Nursing Organizations," of which the American Association of Nurse Anesthetists was a founding member. A loose affiliate of speciality nursing organizations and the American Nurses' Association, the purpose of the Federation is to achieve greater coordination in areas of mutual interest (e.g., continuing education; expanding role of the nurse; licensure and legal aspects of practice; certification; payment for services). Membership is open to nursing organizations that are national in scope, governed by elected bodies, have bylaws defining purposes and functions for improvement of health care, and have a body of knowledge and skill in a defined area of clinical practice. The nurse anesthetists at last had a structure for collegial identity and action.

Geister also noted that because nursing is such intensive work, the tendency can be to emphasize *action* rather than *reflection*—with resultant difficulties. She said, "This preoccupation with *doing* has blurred our understanding of some of the *whys* of our doing—and when we make major moves without such understanding we build up trouble."[36]

In the AANA, it has been the work of Ira Gunn that has provided valuable historical and philosophical contexts in which to consider issues confronting nurse anesthetists. For example, in 1968, in a paper titled "Current Nursing Issues and Their Implications for the Preparation of Nurse Anesthetists," she alerted members to the need for putting an end to the "orphan" image of nurse anesthetists. Declaring, "The nurse anesthetist must establish her identity somewhere if she is to have a progressive future," Gunn asked, "In reality, where do we belong?" She then reflected:

I believe that basic nursing is a prerequisite to anesthesia as we administer it. The opportunities for, and knowledge gained from the study of physiological changes in patients during the [nursing] course are indispensable in the preparation of alert, knowledgeable, safe anesthetists. I believe that the attitudes of compassion, protection, and support of patients fostered in schools of nursing are essential ingredients to the development of responsible, safe anesthetists. I believe that anatomy, physiology and chemistry taught during the course have the potential of an excellent base on which to build our broader and greater knowledge of the human body and its function, as it relates to anesthesia.[37]

In the coming years, Gunn's work would continue to reflect this thinking, defining the nurse anesthetist as the first of a "new breed of nurse, the nurse functioning in an expanded, extended role, before her role in most other specialities was dreamed of, or formalized."[38]

Vietnam

Admitting males to AANA membership was long resisted. In her first Presidential Report (1936), Hilda Salomon called for "some definite action . . . regarding the acceptance of male anesthetists as members in the Association."[39] In the course of her first term, the application of a registered graduate male nurse had been denied by the trustees. Subsequent efforts to change Association bylaws in 1937, 1942, and 1945 were also unsuccessful. Not until 1947 were men permitted to join, and, according to Miriam Shupp, that change was quietly made by her in the midst of members' concern over who would be eligible to take the qualifying examination ("any *person* who"). "Of course Hilda [Salomon] was delighted, because she had been yelling about that for years, that it wasn't fair."[40]

In 1961, the AANA *Bulletin* noted the trend in the United States Army toward increasing the number of men anesthetists. Dubbed "Ethernauts," the first all-male class to complete the year-long course in anesthesiology for nurses at Walter Reed General Hospital, Washington, DC, graduated in May 1961; Letterman General Hospital School of Anesthesia, San Francisco, then graduated an all-male class. The increased training also reflected a greater military need, as involvement in Vietnam deepened.

The role of male nurses in that conflict was unique. As Dr. Richard Redman, RN, has noted, it was "the first war in American history in which professional nurses were drafted as nurses for military service. While nurses have always been involved in U.S. military activities, they had served as volunteers, never as conscripts, until 1966. That tradition was broken when a special draft of male professional nurses was issued by the Department of Defense to meet increased requirements for military personnel during escalation of the Vietnam war. Interestingly, nurses who were women were specifically excluded."[41] Special Call Number 38 produced a total of 151 nurses.[42]

Nurse anesthetists in Vietnam had a special role to play in new approaches to the treatment of the severely wounded. They served on helicopter missions, providing emergency first aid and resuscitation techniques to casualites, many of whom formerly would have died before or during evacuation. Upon arrival at the surgical facility, it was often the nurse anesthetist who became the director of initial or continued resuscitation procedures. As Army Colonel, Ret., John A. Jenicek, described it, in the surgery, as part of "the anesthesia team (physician and/or nurse anesthetist and/or corpsman), [the mission is] to support the circulating volume, the oxygen demand and the anesthetic needs of the patient as well as to treat and correct all abnormal physiological and pharmacological responses of the casualty; all the while providing as near optimal surgical conditions as possible for the equally busy surgical teams." Colonel Jenicek added, "From this trial of supreme skill under fire emerges a new facet of excellence of the nurse anesthetist. Decisions must be instant, instinctively right and based on knowledge and experience. Either as a member of or the leader of such a team, the daily contribution of the nurse anesthetist [male *and* female] to casualty survival has earned professional praise from military and civilian consultants."[43]

David R. Fletcher, CRNA, has recorded the experience of a male nurse anesthetist in Vietnam, 1968, in the following memoir:

I entered the service in 1964 as an Operating Room Nurse and during my first assignment requested and was sent to the Flight Nurse Course in 1965; I received my flight nurse wings upon completion of that course. In 1967, I was accepted and sent to the Nurse Anesthesia Residency Program at Wilford Hall Medical Center, and graduated as an anesthetist in July, 1967. Nine months after graduation from anesthesia school I received my orders to Da Nang Air Base and the 903rd Aeromedical Evacuation Squadron (AMES) as a flight nurse. The detachment at Da Nang had seven nurses (two anesthetists and five general duty) and thirty-two technicians. We were responsible for the evacuation of patients in the I corps of northern South Vietnam.

During my year I participated in 170 + combat missions as a crew member. The aircraft most frequently used was the C130. We did use other types of aircraft depending on the location of the patients and the type of runway available for landing. The type of patients we were called to transport varied from stabilized to triage needing further care not available at the triage area. The crew caring for the patients on these flights was one flight nurse and two medical technicians. The capacity on a C130 is 50 litters and approximately 40 ambulatory patients or a combination of the two.

At times we were called to evacuate Vietnamese patients from some small provincial hospital and operate out of dirt runways with minimal information about the type of patients to expect, and often not sure of the numbers involved or how many family members to expect. These flights were generally back to Da Nang to the larger hospital for more long-term care.

During my year in Vietnam, the Squadron and all of its operating locations evacuated approximately 50,000 patients. These patients were transported to various hospitals in Vietnam; only very few patients were transported out of country. The out-of-country patient movement was done by MAC (Military Airlift Command), and involved the movement of patients to Japan and back to the States.

Some of our anesthetists worked in the forward area at the CSF (casualty staging facilities) and helped prepare the patients for transport once the aircraft arrived.

During my tour I was awarded the Air Medal with 4 Oak Leaf Clusters, the Bronze Star, and the Distinguished Flying Cross. I received the Distinguished Flying Cross for evacuating a 125-bed hospital in the side winds of a typhoon that was approaching the coast of Vietnam. Two of the patients with head injuries stopped breathing after take-off, and I had to use my anesthesia training to ventilate the patients with Ambu bags until we arrived at Da Nang and they could be transported to the hospital and placed on ventilators.

At times we were called to evacuate patients from areas close to the battle area and would be under fire while loading patients. There were times when the aircraft was hit by ground fire, and I guess by luck no one was hurt or hit.

A day's work was often sixteen to eighteen hours. Some days you would start at noon with an assigned mission and follow the set mission and end when the mission ended. Other days you were on call and did emergency flights when a call came. This type of flight might be to a provincial hospital or it might be a critical patient who needed care at a special hospital. Or it might be a battle that was occurring and they needed patients transported to hospitals. We had a standing rule to transport all individuals no matter their condition because they had no chance in the field and their only hope was at a larger medical facility.

We had nurse anesthetists in Vietnam as early as 1965, some in a civilian status. Others served during the early years of Vietnam when the female [Air Force] anesthetist and nurses were not yet allowed in the country. As an aside, our squadron had thirty-one or thirty-two nurses, and only one was female during the year that I was stationed there. That was because when loading the aircraft we all helped to place litters inside, and it was very heavy work. That is not to say some females could not have done the job. It is only saying that it was the reason behind the decision.[44]

It is important to note that the Army, Navy, and Air Force had different policies regarding female nurse anesthetists.

Another view of Vietnam is presented by Patricia L. Walsh, CRNA, in *Forever Sad the Hearts*. It is a powerful novel based on her fourteen months' service as a volunteer in a civilian hospital established by the US Agency for International Development. It provides other insights into the nurse anesthetist experience. For example, in hitching a ride to Da Nang, Kate Shea introduces herself to the pilot, who has invited her to sit beside him:

> "A nurse, huh?" he said, pulling the curtain back across the door.
> "A nurse anesthetist," I corrected. "I put people to sleep for surgery."
> "I thought doctors did that."
> "They do, but anesthetists do the same thing. Sometimes we work together, sometimes we work alone." He was nodding as if he understood, but I was used to the confusion my job title always produced. "Anesthetists are R.N.s with two years of additional training in anesthesia," I explained. "Anesthesiologists are physicians."
> "And I thought you were a little doughnut dollie," he said with a smile.
> "A what?"
> "Doughnut dollie—Red Cross. They go up to Da Nang sometimes."
> "Are they nurses?"
> "No; none I've ever met, anyway. They're called doughnut dollies because of the doughnuts and coffee they sell."

In another passage, in the operating room, Kate asks: "Why don't we have any anesthesiologists over here?" reflecting,

> It wasn't uncommon for nurse anesthetists to work alone, but the severity of injuries we encountered, coupled with the complication of anesthetizing anemic tuberculosis victims, should certainly have qualified us for physician consultation.
> "Are you kidding?" Shelly laughed. "I've never even seen one volunteer for the AMA's two-month program."
> "I guess they prefer nicer climates," I said.
> "Preferably with no bullets in the air," she said.
> I'd been out of school only a short time, and already I'd learned that nurse anesthetists were considered incompetent in places like Denver or San Francisco, but completely qualified to do anything and everything in the inner city slums or isolated small towns. I remarked quietly on this to Shelly, who nodded her head in agreement.
> "Our competence is also related to the setting and rising of the sun," she said, not bothering to lower her voice in the presence of

Dr. Ramirez. "As the sun goes down, we become proportionately more capable of handling anything that comes along. By three A.M., we're goddamned miracle workers."

"You girls are a couple of cynics," Jim Ramirez said.

"We're just tired of making those bastards rich while we do the work," Shelly said.

"There are some good ones," I said. "I learned a lot from the ones at the hospital where I trained, and we all got along fine."

"Not where I trained," she said. "Half of them weren't board-certified and could barely speak English. All they knew how to do was count, one thousand dollars, two thousand dollars."[45]

Nurse anesthetists also contributed to patient care in the Vietnam experience through the development of new field equipment. Jenicek noted that anesthesia equipment "had not been changed in the field units since World War II. The Cuban incident briefly mobilized the equipment and fleetingly exposed its antiquity and inadequacy, but the field chests were closed again before any significant changes were made, although many were actually initiated based on communications received from nurse anesthetists on the scene."[46] By July 1967 a new field anesthesia machine was standardized and in place in all active hospital units in Vietnam. The new machine—smaller and lighter than the 1939 model—had an increased carbon dioxide absorbing cannister, and could supply ether, nitrous oxide, cyclopropane, methoxyflurane, halothane, and oxygen or air for anesthesia as needed. A new field anesthesia chest was also in place, one that could provide the anesthetist with about three days' worth of supplies. The army nurse anesthetists made significant contributions to the design of this unit.

Of the ten nurses who lost their lives in the Vietnam conflict, two were nurse anesthetists: First Lieutenant Kenneth R. Shoemaker, Jr., CRNA, and First Lieutenant Jerome Edwin Olmsted, CRNA. Both were assigned to the 67th Evacuation Hospital at Qui Nhon, and were killed in the crash of a C-47 transport plane carrying wounded from Pleiku to Qui Nhon. Their names were included in Washington's Vietnam Veteran Memorial.

ASA-AANA: Years of Dialogue

Not since 1947 had there been any communication between the American Society of Anesthesiologists and the American Association of Nurse Anesthetists—not since the ASA's Board of Directors adopted the "anti-Adriani" resolution, prohibiting the participation of its members in the anesthesia education of any persons other than doctors of medicine. Beginning in the mid-1950s, Presidents of the ASA began calling for a new study of the field of anesthesiology, including practice, research and teaching. President Albert M. Betcher launched the undertaking in 1963. It was to be conducted by an outside agency, so that the results would be "fresh" and "unbiased."[47]

After the pilot study was completed, Dr. Robert D. Dripps, chairman of the Advisory Committee, said, "Outsiders . . . have recognized many things which we have known about, but have in a sense ignored, hoping I suppose that 'they would go away'!"[48] If one of those "things" were nurse anesthetists, it is clear why they *could* not go away. Surveys of anesthesia service conducted by the AANA show that it was nurse anesthetists who were providing the majority of anesthesia care in the United States:[49]

	1955	1965	1971
1. Members of the AANA	34%	46%	48.5%
2. Members of the ASA	18	39	38.34
3. Physicians whose qualifications as specialists are unknown	27	11	9.7
4. Nurses whose qualifications are unknown	19	3	2.8
5. Neither registered nurses nor physicians	2	1	0.66

According to Betcher, it was, in fact, the present and projected personnel needs in the field that caused the ASA to "initiate efforts to establish relations with certified nurse anesthetists."[50]

Thus, in 1963, Betcher, as president of the ASA, unofficially contacted AANA President Mary Alice Costello to investigate the possibility of a dialogue between the two organizations. Her response could not be a surprise to anyone familiar with the history of the nurse anesthetist experience. Much damage had been done, and could not be expected to be quickly repaired: "The question that we discussed has been brought before the officers of this association on several occasions and we have been individually approached on the same subject. With 11,526 members in the association, many of whom have been subjected over the years to quite opposite attitudes from the one that is now proposed, it may take many years before the Board of Trustees could adopt the suggestions that have been made. This is not to say that we will not watch every avenue by which we will continue to cooperate in all matters that pertain to patient welfare."[51]

In 1964 the ASA House of Delegates voted to permit members to participate in the teaching of anesthesia to registered nurses, thus rescinding the seventeen-year-old "Anti-Adriani Bylaw." The same year, an ASA/AANA Liaison Committee was formed, and the first joint meeting between the organizations' officers was held in 1966. To facilitate the discussion of this committee, participant Dr. John Adriani asked AANA Executive Director Florence McQuillen to prepare a statement reflecting what the Association would want from an improved relationship with the ASA.[52] Again, given the history of the organizational relationship, it is not surprising that the AANA viewed as essential the maintenance of the Association's autonomy, a guarantee of "no interference with the progress of the educational programs of the Association," and a curbing of anti-nurse anesthetist activity and publicity.[53]

A story in *Time* magazine of November 5, 1965, "Anesthesiology," that focused on the annual ASA meeting, and contained the observation that "Nearly gone is the nurse-technician who dates back to the early days of ether and chloroform and whose only function was to render the patient insensitive to pain," was reminiscent of the postwar anti–nurse anesthetist publicity campaign. On this occasion, however, ASA President John J. Bonica called AANA Executive Director Mc-Quillen to express concern over the reporter's misunderstanding, and to assure her that the official stand of the ASA was one of wanting to cooperate with nurse anesthetists. McQuillen reported that she "assured him that we do not wear shoes that do not fit and do not classify ourselves as anesthesia technicians but that I could not guarantee that some members may react violently against what appears to be a renewed onslaught against the nurse anesthetists."[54]

In January 1968 a statement affirming the desirability of continued cooperation between the American Society of Anesthesiologists and the American Association of Nurse Anesthetists was published jointly in the bulletins of the two Associations. It recommended that "close liaisons be developed between these organizations for enhancing the quality and quantity of available personnel, for advancing educational opportunities, for determining ethical relationships and for the overall improvement of patient care."[55] Each group extended to the other a growing number of invitations to attend clinical sessions on local, state, and national levels. Each association also stressed that this did not include the right to be present at business or committee meetings of the other group. An anesthesiologist speakers' bureau was made available for use in AANA educational programs. In 1970, the ASA-AANA Joint Committee issued a statement calling attention of all members to the cooperative policies, noting that "it is the desire of

these organizations to work closely together in order to accomplish
. . . the overall improvement of patient care."[56]

Finally, in 1972, an ASA-AANA Joint Statement on Anesthesia
Practice was issued. It was of considerable significance because it
recognized the Certified Registered Nurse Anesthetist as an appropriate anesthesia care provider, and it acknowledged that "the ideal
circumstances of qualified anesthesiologists and nurse anesthetists
working together as an anesthesia care team may not be totally possible in the future."[57] The statement seemed to promise a new relationship of collegiality between the two anesthesia provider groups.

But the apparent rapprochement would be short-lived.

The End of an Era

The 1970s was a period of reform. Just as the nation went through
the process of seeing to the replacement of its leader, Richard M.
Nixon, the American Association of Nurse Anesthetists had decided
at long last to replace the person who had led the organization
through difficult times (the consensus is that it was she who single-
handedly held together the entire structure), but whose solitary management style had lost its effectiveness. In a spirit of reform, then, the
elected leaders saw to it that the appointed one resigned in 1970.
Florence A. McQuillen—"Mac"—stepped down from her active post
as Executive Director, and became "Director Emeritus." President
Virginia A. Gaffey gave one perspective to the situation when she
observed,

> This year saw the end of an era for our Association. Miss Florence
> McQuillen has worked tirelessly, diligently, conscientiously, and pa-
> tiently for the cause of the AANA. Seven days a week, as many
> hours as needed in a day, she has labored since 1948 in our behalf.
> Four years ago she told the Board of Trustees of her hope to retire.
> Now it is time for her to retire and to do the many things that she
> has been postponing for years until she no longer had the Associa-
> tion's activities as a full-time activity.[58]

There were difficulties following Mac's "retirement." Just as
Hodgins had attempted to continue to run Association activities from
her hospital room at Lakeside, so, too, did McQuillen continue her
efforts. Goldie Brangman, AANA President 1973–74, recalled:

> She insisted on coming to the office every day, every day, and she
> was supposed to be preparing a history of something or other, but

she was still running the office. And nobody understood the problem, and that's when it got sticky.[59]

And, like Hodgins, Mac, too, had "resentment" "directed toward the 'then' people."

As Brangman noted, McQuillen "never delegated any authority. There was absolutely, positively no delegation of authority." "Mac did a great job when she came in, because the office was in shambles. And Mac built it up. But, then, unfortunately. . . ."[60]

The "unfortunate" part was that, under McQuillen's controlling personality, powerful intellect, and personal presence, the Association's structure had become inverted:

> While it was the Board of Directors' business to tell the staff, "This is what we'd like to see done, now you get busy and implement it," the staff members were making the decisions and then telling the Board of Directors it had been done.[61]

McQuillen was a paradoxical figure. In her first year as executive director, she reminded members that "we [in the executive office] do not set policies: that is done for us by you and your duly elected Board of Trustees. We do hope to carry out your assignments."[62] Telling members that "the Executive Office is essentially the workshop for the Association," she duly focused her yearly Report on the *quantity* of material processed by her office. For example, in 1963, she reported 697,517 addressograph impressions made, 44,529 pieces of first class mail sent, 4,699 changes of address recorded, and 1,524 parcel post packages sent (totaling 4,411 pounds).[63] Yet, at the same time, McQuillen in fact controlled the flow of information in the Association. Under Mac, the *Journal* became a vehicle chiefly for clinical studies, and the *Bulletin* (which was begun in 1947) a report of activities of members and state affiliates. The Association publications ceased to communicate, much less discuss, controversial, critical issues. Similarly, Mac herself produced the minutes of the meetings of the Board of Trustees, thus controlling the record of business. She also prepared the agenda for board meetings, and, as Mary Alice Costello, president 1963–64, recalled, "she wouldn't give us the agenda beforehand. So, when you were President, an issue would come up, and you would have to say, 'Miss McQuillen, would you explain this to the Board?' because you didn't know about it. And she didn't want anybody to know about it."[64] Goldie Brangman described her experience as treasurer: "I would fly in [to Chicago] from New York and spend most of the time sitting in the hall crocheting, while I waited to be called in. . . . I was handed a piece of paper to stand up and read, a report that had been written for me, Mac's report. . . . If you had asked me what the assets were, in no way could I have told you, because I didn't know. And I didn't know any way to find out, because Miss McQuillen was not going to tell me—treasurer or no treasurer." Brangman rebelled and became "a little unpopular with Mac" when she recommended that the treasurer become part of the board and be given a vote.[65]

McQuillen not only controlled Association affairs, kept count of every piece of mail and penny of postage, answered her own phone, and performed tasks such as folding papers for the examination program, she also edited *Anesthesia Abstracts*—a dramatic intellectual achievement and major contribution to the field of anesthesia. Begun in 1937 by Dr. John S. Lundy, it originally represented the work of the Journal Club of the Section of Anesthesiology at Mayo Clinic. Those meetings did not continue, and the project shortly became the solitary effort of McQuillen. Though this massive scholarly undertaking bore the names of both Lundy and McQuillen (with the doctor's name given precedence) it was, as Lundy later said, all her work. McQuillen finally gave up *Anesthesia Abstracts* in 1965, and it ceased publication. That same year, Lundy said of McQuillen and this enterprise,

> Very likely she is now the best-read person on the literature of anesthesia. Her contribution to the development of the literature on anesthesia is not excelled and probably will not be.[66]

There is no doubt that McQuillen possessed formidable intellectual stature. She contended with the hostilities of organized anesthesiologists and enjoyed long friendships with leading figures like Lundy and Adriani. She was uniquely suited to lead nurse anesthetists through years of turbulent challenge and growth.

Mac was also a woman who "liked a good drink and good food and a good story," a woman with a "big heart" who was "almost motherly" to her staff. Large in mind *and* body, she related a telling childhood memory to Costello. The latter recalled,

> She used to tell me that when she was a little girl, she was always heavy. And she wouldn't get invited to parties. But her mother used to tell her that God made people fat because they needed a big heart. And she had a big heart.[67]

For her own part, McQuillen, in sketching a brief review of her twenty-two-year tenure as executive director, highlighted the successful accreditation program; the creation of the Council (which increased participation of state affiliates and was the forerunner of the

Assembly of States); the adoption in 1969 of an optional continuing education program (which became mandatory in 1977); and the growth of the membership, from 3,200 to 14,539.[68] Her last words in this "Director Emeritus" report—"I believe that the members should have what they want but it should be arrived at by the democratic process of the majority decision being accepted by all members"— seem unintentionally ironic, given her manner of conducting Association affairs. On the other hand, there is no mistaking the intentional irony in her last "From the Plaza" column:

> This column is the last that will appear over the signature of Florence A. McQuillen as Executive Director. . . .
>
> In assuming the title of Director Emeritus it was necessary to explain to some of the members of the staff the role that each person would assume when the many changes take place. To this end we asked members of the staff to look up the various words, among them the words Executive and Emeritus. The definition best suited to our use of the word Executive was any person or body charged with administrative or executive work.
>
> The dictionary gives a choice for the word Emeritus. It describes Emeritus as "retired from office or active duty on account of age, infirmity or long and faithful service and honored with nonofficial position and title corresponding to those held."
>
> The title "Consultant to the Board of Trustees" could have many ramifications. . . . [Elsewhere] it was pointed out that one of the unwritten rules in the management consulting business is to wear a hat but the hat must not have a feather. . . .
>
> In this new capacity as Director Emeritus-Consultant, I will still be in touch with you. As has been called to my attention by members, they have known no other Executive Director. This is true of more than 8000 of the members.

Mac concluded with the benediction, "In putting on the new, feather-less hat, I can only wish for my successor the same kindness and consideration that you have shown to me during these years."[69]

· 7 ·

A Return to Roots

I n her 1974 year-end President's Report, Goldie D. Brangman addressed the effects of the major negative legacy of McQuillen's years: a lack of communication within the Association. Brangman's words provide an interesting glimpse of the experience of many members as the years of Mac's long tenure wore on:

> Obviously, when members have little or no part in establishing policies or in making decisions, they feel little responsibility for them; and the effectiveness of any national strategy or plan is seriously compromised, since it will not have major support at the member level.
>
> Then too, when members are excluded from the decision-making process, a fertile field is provided for rumors—rumors which spread easily, eroding the confidence of the members in their association and decreasing the potential effectiveness of the organization.
>
> Even more important, such exclusion leads to the practice of withholding information, making it difficult to level with members when actions, following decisions made at the top, are reported to them—particularly if the actions have resulted in faulty or inadequate operations.
>
> The members, on the other hand, tend to compound the problem by becoming frustrated, apathetic, or inhibited. Many, feeling that nothing they suggest or report will be acted upon, simply stop communicating entirely and refuse to become involved at any level in the organization. The end result of this abdication of responsibility is that it is left to others to function, without any need for accountability, since even this is not demanded by the members. There may be advantages to this system, but I believe they are totally outweighed by the resulting distrust, disinterest, and disenchantment of many members with the organization.

Brangman continued by stressing the need for member involvement in all phases of the Association. In her call for participation,

Brangman echoed the Association leaders of the 1930s, during the formative years of the national group:

> Improving the internal communication system of an organization is not always easy. The national organization must first face its responsibility for keeping the state officers, and through them, the members, continually and completely informed. By this, I do not mean simply informing members of decisions made and actions taken by the Board and implemented by the Executive Staff. It is not enough for the Board and the Executive Staff alone to understand the current mix of needs. The more widespread this knowledge, the more effectively members can contribute to seeing that policies and priorities make sense.
>
> An effective organization continually looks for ways to involve members in the development of plans, policies, and procedures on a year-round basis, because through participation comes understanding, and members can then, as a rule, wholeheartedly support the interim decisions and actions of their Board.[1]

Brangman and the other post-McQuillen leaders clearly understood that a return to that earlier spirit was essential if increasingly complex challenges to the profession were successfully to be met. The transition, however, was not without casualties.

A Matter of Professional Autonomy

The nation's economic recession, energy crisis, inflation, weariness with the continued involvement in Vietnam—all contributed to an era in which reform and change were fairly well-mandated. President Nixon referred to a "health care crisis" and launched a decade of questioning about the entire field, putting an end to a period of postwar growth of social entitlements. As Paul Starr has observed, "Practitioners, hospitals, researchers, and medical schools [had] enjoyed a broad grant of authority to run their own affairs. In the 1970s this mandate ran out. . . . Rising costs brought medical care under more critical scrutiny, and the federal government, as a major buyer of health services, intervened in unprecedented ways."[2]

Revised criteria for nationally recognized accrediting agencies and associations were published by the US Commissioner of Education, of the Department of Health, Education and Welfare on January 16, 1969. These criteria superseded those previously in effect. To obtain renewal of its status as the accrediting agency for schools of anesthesia, the AANA acted to comply with the new regulations, published in final form in 1974. Thus, in 1975, separate Councils on Accreditation, Certification, and Practice were formed. (When continuing education became mandatory in 1977, the Council on Recertification was created.) Affiliated with the AANA and remaining under its corporate structure, the councils nevertheless were given complete autonomy— the major concern of the government agency. As a further assurance of independence, membership on the councils included certified registered nurse anesthetists (CRNAs), anesthesiologists and other members of the medical profession, hospital administrators, representatives of other relevant agencies, and the public itself.

It will be recalled that several years of ASA-AANA dialogue, initiated at the request of the physician group, culminated in the 1972 Joint Statement on Anesthesia Practice. It had seemed to augur a new period of cooperation. Yet, the government process of review and revision of accrediting agencies provided an opportunity for physicians to attempt to take control of the nurse anesthetist profession. And the Joint Statement would be used by the anesthesiologists to justify their activities.

The first such action occurred in 1970–72, involving an ASA Anesthesia Manpower Study, supported by a grant from the Health Manpower Division, HEW. The AANA was requested to furnish its membership list as a basis for assessing the demography of both nurse anesthetists and anesthesiologists. When completed, the study's cover sheet stated that it had been performed in cooperation with the AANA. The implication was that the AANA was in agreement with its conclusions and recommendations, whereas, in fact, the AANA had not been asked to comment on the study methodology, the analysis of the data, or the conclusions drawn by the ASA Manpower Committee. (One such objection would be to the fact that, while the study was limited to actively practicing CRNAs, the data relative to anesthesiologists included active, retired, and residents in training.) The last paragraph of the study stated:

> While anesthesiologists are involved to some extent in teaching the nurse in anesthesia at the local level, physicians provide minimal input into standards of accreditation of approved schools, curriculum, and the certification of nurse anesthetists. Both the American Society of Anesthesiologists and the American Association of Nurse Anesthetists in a joint statement [published in January, 1972] agreed that "the ideal circumstances" for the delivery of quality anesthesia care is to have "qualified anesthesiologists and nurse anesthetists working together as an anesthesia care team."

Against the background of this agreement, the conclusion was then drawn:

An important step in achieving this goal, which appears to be in the best interest of patient care, is to provide for more direct involvement of the anesthesiologists in the establishment of policy relative to accreditation, curriculum, certification, and quality assurance for the nurse involved in anesthesia care.

Ira Gunn noted that "ASA representatives took this recommendation to the Office of Education and began working with that Office in an attempt to gain greater control over nurse anesthetist education and accreditation. The first AANA knew of this was when representatives of the USOE [United States Office of Education] called AANA to set up a meeting between representatives of ASA, AANA, and USOE."[3] The AANA filed a formal protest with the Bureau of Health Manpower.

In other actions, members of the American Society of Anesthesiologists, acting within the framework of the ASA Ad Hoc Committee on the Anesthesia Health Care Team, challenged the legitimacy of the AANA accreditation program before the United States Office of Education and the Council on Postsecondary Accreditation (COPA). The hearings on the AANA's petition for continued recognition as the accrediting agency for schools and programs of nurse anesthesia were conducted on March 12, 1975, before Subcommittee III of the National Advisory Committee on Accreditation and Institutional Eligibility, US Office of Education. Some 100 CRNAs, fifteen anesthesiologists, and representatives from the American Nurses' Association, the American College of Nurse Midwives, and the Association of Operating Room Nurses were in attendance.

The ASA committee charged the AANA with noncompliance of specific US Department of Health, Education and Welfare (HEW) criteria. The ASA committee argued that anesthesiologists should have equal representation with nurse anesthetists in any accrediting mechanism for nurse anesthesia programs. In response to a question from a committeeman, the anesthesiologists replied that they did not feel that a 50 percent representation would, in fact, give them control of the accreditation council.

The Project Manager for the AANA Petition, Gunn, argued that AANA structural changes and proposed bylaw revisions did comply with HEW criteria. Further, she insisted that "while the American Association of Nurse Anesthetists fully concurs in the inclusion of the public and the community of interest into decision making relative to accreditation, we do believe that the ultimate responsibility for quality assurance for education and practice of nurse anesthetists should rest with nurse anesthetists."[4]

Her sentiments were in accord with those of Dr. Pearl Dunkley, Deputy Executive Director of the American Nurses' Association. Dunkley's words before the subcommittee were of great significance, not the least because they signaled once again the strengthening ties between nurse anesthetists and other nurses, a sense of the need for solidarity among *all* nursing groups. Dunkley stated that "it is nursing's position that each profession bears the ultimate responsibility for its own quality assurance (education and practice), while providing for input and consideration for the ever-broadening community of interest within which each profession exists." She added (in language that recalled the Dagmar Nelson case) that "since the legal basis for the practice of the nurse anesthetist derives from the nurse practice acts of each state, and not the medical practice acts, the nurse anesthetist is a nurse specialist, not a physician expander, extender, or assistant."[5]

Dr. E. S. Siker, an ASA past president and member of the ASA Ad Hoc Committee on the Anesthesia Health Care Team, informed Subcommittee III that some anesthesiologists were proposing an alternative—and competitive—approach to the accreditation of nurse anesthesia programs. Known as the Faculty of Nurse Anesthesia Schools (FNAS), this physician-designed structure did allow representation of one anesthesiologist and one CRNA member per school/program. However, as Gunn pointed out, "since a significant proportion of the CRNAs were employees of the anesthesiologist or anesthesiologist group," this plan would have, in fact, placed control of nurse anesthesia in the hands of the anesthesiologists.[6] FNAS also planned its own nurse anesthetist certification program.

In January 1976 the AANA Board of Directors published a policy statement expressing concern over the physician-sponsored (FNAS) accreditation program for nurse anesthetists, and reaffirmed "its commitment to the following position on the credentialing of professionals and in particular that of nurse anesthetists":

1. Individual professions must assume primary responsibility for quality assurance mechanisms relative to their membership while providing for adequate input from the community of interest and the public.

   a. The AANA Council structure provides the appropriate bodies for administering the accreditation and certification programs and makes provision for input by anesthesiologists, hospital administrators, nurse anesthesia students and the public as well as the nurse anesthesia profession.

   b. The AANA Council on Accreditation, by virtue of its approval by the Office of Education, U.S. Department of Health, Education and Welfare has shown itself to be in compliance with all government regulations pertaining to nationally recognized accrediting agencies.

2. The Association of Faculty of Nurse Anesthesia Schools (FNAS) is neither representative of historical precedence, professional tradition, nor recognized by the Office of Education, U.S. Department of Health, Education and Welfare and has no experience in the accreditation of nurse anesthesia educational programs and certification of nurse anesthetists.

3. Membership by individuals in the FNAS organization is by individual choice with no constraints for membership imposed by that organization's bylaws and cannot be construed as implying AANA approval, endorsement or participation.

4. AANA will not abdicate its professional responsibilities for credentialing but stands ready to participate in and/or support its Councils' participation in dialogue aimed at increased cooperation and collaboration with any group which has as its primary purpose and intent the improvement of professional services to the public. This especially includes our physician colleagues in Anesthesiology.[7]

The failure to challenge successfully the AANA's position as the accrediting agency for nurse anesthesia programs probably caused the abandonment of the anesthesiologist-sponsored accreditation and certification programs for nurse anesthetists. The abandonment may also have been in part a result of the ASA being the object of Federal Trade Commission and Department of Justice actions challenging some of its own practices. For example, in December, 1975, the Federal Trade Commission (which had begun monitoring the hearings before USOE and COPA) initiated an inquiry into the American Society of Anesthesiologists' ethical guidelines regarding salaried arrangements with hospitals. In June 1978 the ASA House of Delegates in a special meeting voted to accept a proposed settlement of that investigation that prohibited the ASA from restraining anesthesiologists in practice other than a fee-for-service basis. A 1975 Department of Justice civil antitrust suit against the ASA, alleging a conspiracy to "raise, fix, stabilize and maintain fees" charged by its members, resulted in a two-week trial. On June 22, 1979, the court ordered the government suit dismissed, finding that the ASA's Relative Value Guide did not violate antitrust laws.[8]

The increasingly strained relations between the AANA and ASA caused by the latter's challenge to the AANA's status as accrediting agency for nurse anesthesia schools and programs were exacerbated by the 1975 AANA move to obtain support for third-party reimbursement legislation for nurse anesthetists. AANA Executive Director

Bernice Baum, in conjunction with the AANA Washington consultant and the Board of Directors, submitted a policy proposal to Senator Herman E. Talmadge, Chairman of the House Ways and Means Committee. In her August 12, 1975, letter to Talmadge, Baum had indicated that there was no evidence of a difference in the quality of anesthesia care between nurse anesthetists and physicians. According to one writer, "It was factual that no data existed to prove a difference . . ., however, it was also true that this statement not only threatened the authority structure of anesthesiologists but also insulted them. . . . The Baum letter caused open warfare from local through national levels of the anesthesia community. The more aggressive and chauvinistic nurse anesthetists applauded Baum's action. Those who deferred to anesthesiologists, whose employment was dependent upon anesthesiologists, or who believed in the superiority of anesthesiologists were infuriated."[9]

The AANA-ASA Liaison Committee met in December 1975 and "unanimously pledged their support of further cooperation" between the two groups, in spite of the "serious deterioration" in relationships between the organizations. The January, 1976, *AANA News Bulletin* reported of that meeting:

> It was explained that in approaching Senator Talmadge's committee, the AANA's efforts were directed politically to get recognition for CRNAs as purveyors of anesthesia care by third-party payers. The AANA was seeking for its members compensation on an equitable basis; its actions were not aimed at denigrating the anesthesiologist or interfering with his economic relationship. Furthermore, the AANA representatives stated, the AANA intends to maintain the professional relationship now existing and continue to progress toward the concept of the anesthesia care team.[10]

Even the American Medical Association seemed intent on helping smooth the troubled situation with a *JAMA* editorial, "Cooperation and Educational Efforts Lead to Better Service," by Senior Editor, Dr. Z. Danilevicius (April 21, 1975). It reflected that "Two most important factors helping to provide the best possible anesthetic services in the United States are cordial cooperation between the anesthesiologists and the nurse anesthetists, and the sincere effort to improve education and scientific sophistication of the nurse-anesthetist."[11]

However, in March 1976 the ASA Board of Directors withdrew support of the 1972 ASA-AANA Joint Statement on Anesthesia Practice, and embraced a different definition of the Anesthesia Care Team. This one put the anesthesiologist in a leadership position.

That spring, the AANA Executive Director resigned. In a real sense, McQuillen's farewell "blessing" upon her successor had proven efficacious. . . .

A Matter of Control

In a February 1976 essay in the *AANA Journal,* Dr. Jeffrey A. Brown summarized the central issue in the ASA-AANA conflict:

> Your rights to control anesthetist training, conduct peer review, help define client needs, and secure what you consider to be an acceptable level of reimbursement are no mean rights. They are the foundation of your professional autonomy, your right to control your work. The ability to exercise this right is what some sociologists say is really what makes professionals differ from nonprofessionals.

He added, "It, therefore is very understandable why some of you worry about the future of nurse anesthesia as a profession."[12]

In her important study, *"The Physician's Hand": Work Culture and Conflict in American Nursing,* Barbara Melosh has questioned whether nursing itself *is* a profession because, "within the existing division of labor, . . . nurses' autonomy is constrained by medicine's professional dominance."[13] Nurse anesthetists, nursing's first clinical specialty, have been on the cutting edge of this issue for decades. After first winning the legal right to exist, they have since insisted on their right to self-definition and self-determination. Given the deeply entrenched cultural dominance of medicine over nursing (rooted in that of male over female), this is a much more formidable struggle.

Gunn has noted the nurse anesthetists' "increased security in a legitimate nursing role," as well as "the rapprochement between nursing and nurse anesthesia."[14] She has also articulated the fundamental differences between medicine's perception of the nurse anesthetist and the latter's self-definition:

> Basically, the philosophy of practice of the two groups is incompatible with merger as envisioned by anesthesiologists. Their view of the nurse anesthetist is that of a physician's assistant, while most nurse anesthetists perceive themselves as nurse specialists. The difference in these views is that the anesthesiologist sees the nurse anesthetist as being a physician extender, helping him to do more work, while being dependent upon him in all aspects of practice.
>
> The nurse specialist view is one in which the nurse anesthetist provides anesthesiological services to a patient as an agent of a physician, any physician, while providing nursing services to that

same patient and holding independent professional responsibility for those nursing services. In this role, the nurse anesthetist may consult with an anesthesiologist (or with other physicians) as may be indicated, or refer the patient through the patient's primary physician to an anesthesiologist if patient requirement warrants such referral.

In fact, as a philosophical construct, the practice of anesthesia is neither exclusively medical nor exclusively nursing, though it more nearly fits into the nursing model of the care process than it does into the medical model of the cure process. Anesthesia is a procedure or a process through which patients are rendered insensitive to pain, and in many instances, paralyzed for purposes of facilitating diagnosis and/or treatment.

By rendering the patient incapable of providing care for himself, the anesthetist must become the care provider—and this care is basically nursing. However, in those instances where the patient's health status and the magnitude of the surgery predisposes him to requirements for a predominance of medical judgment, the care provided is medical in nature. Dr. Meyer Saklad, a prominent anesthesiologist, has stated that, "The number of medical judgments made by the anesthesiologist in any single [anesthetic] administration are few indeed." Therefore, anesthesia, as a specialty, can appropriately fit into both medicine and nursing.[15]

The magnitude of the difficulty in achieving what one *AANA News Bulletin* headlined, "Cooperation, communication, and coexistence: Is it attainable?" is made clear by contrasting Gunn's 1975 statement above with that of ASA President, Dr. John W. Ditzler, in his 1976 "President's Annual Report." Detzler declared that anesthesiologists "must especially seek to be the unquestioned dominant force in appropriate patient care, evidenced in every single anesthetic administered in this country. A pragmatist looking at the problems of manpower and of recruitment within the physician specialty believes, and I think correctly, that our traditional concept of one-to-one will require a pluralistic approach and *we* had better set the guidelines (not HEW, AANA, etc.). *We* had better determine how these people will be trained, how their schools will be accredited, how their graduates will be certified, and when and under what circumstances patients may be best served by their graduates when rendering an anesthetic in the absence of a physician, such as in remote and deprived areas. As things now stand, we have competing organizations, not cooperating organizations."[16] (original emphasis)

The AANA's first male (and youngest) president, later executive director, also addressed the issue of "control." In 1977, John Garde

observed, "Many activities of the AANA on the legislative and credentialing fronts have been viewed by certain members of the ASA with
suspicion and sometimes hostility. Many anesthesiologists, like their
colleagues in other medical specialties, believe that the physician is the
controller of the health care team, and as such, should control education, credentialing, quality assurance, and the practice field. There is
little question that current legislation, both at the state and federal
level, as well as the Joint Commission on Accreditation of Hospitals
(JCAH) standards, reflect this view. The word 'control' is unacceptable to nurse anesthetists as a group, as it is to other nurses. . . .
Attempts are being made at both AANA and ASA organizational
levels to decrease tensions, but both groups must recognize that there
are philosophical differences which preclude compromise on all issues. The goal of the CRNA is for the physician groups to recognize
the nurse as a colleague and co-team member, rather than as a
physician assistant or extender."[17] Achievement of that goal would be
momentous for all of nursing.

In fact, some blamed the increasing presence of males in the AANA
for what they perceived to be the Association's failure to accept its
appropriate place in the order of things. The AANA's long-time
friend and supporter, Dr. John Adriani, was one who was especially
angry with its leadership on this count, and cited the growing number
of men from the military services as a major reason for its bad
attitude. Thus, he eventually withdrew his support for the ASA-
AANA Joint Statement on Anesthesia Practice, saying he regretted his
part in its formulation because it conferred a collegial status on nurses
to which they had no right.[18]

Continued Achievement of the AANA

In spite of the challenges and conflicts, the Association continued to
grow. By 1981, there were 20,363 members. There was also a permanent home for the AANA; the Park Ridge, Illinois, building was
purchased in 1978.

That year also saw the beginning of what has come to be known as
"The International Federation of Nurse Anesthetists" (IFNA). Two
European nurse anesthetists attended the AANA annual meeting in
Detroit. One of them, Hermi Lohnert, Switzerland, inquired of Presi-
dent Ronald F. Caulk, CRNA, whether the Association would be
willing to support an international symposium for nurse anesthetists.
Caulk noted, "Of course, the AANA agreed." (Ironically, an invitation
from Finland for cooperation, extended to the Association during the
McCarthy 1950s was rejected: there was a fear of being lured into a
communist enterprise.)[19]

In 1985, the First International Symposium was held in Lucerne, Switzerland. Approximately 250 nurse anesthetists from eleven countries attended. In 1988, the Second International Congress of Nurse Anesthetists was held in Amsterdam; it was attended by 511 nurse anesthetists from sixteen countries. Interest in an international organization was widespread, and a planning meeting was held in Switzerland in September 1988. There resulted agreement on a name, "The International Federation of Nurse Anesthetists," as well as objectives and functions of the new group.

The objectives developed and agreed upon were:

(1) To promote cooperation between nurse anesthetists internationally
(2) To develop and promote educational standards in the field of nurse anesthesia
(3) To develop and promote standards of practice in the field of nurse anesthesia
(4) To provide opportunities for continuing education in anesthesia
(5) To assist nurse anesthetists' associations to improve the standards of nurse anesthesia and the competence of nurse anesthetists
(6) To promote the recognition of nurse anesthesia
(7) To establish and maintain effective cooperation between nurse anesthetists, anesthesiologists and other members of the medical profession, hospitals and agencies representing a community of interest in nurse anesthesia.

The functions adopted were:

(1) To promote continual high quality of patient care
(2) To serve as the authoritative voice of nurse anesthetists and nurse anesthesia internationally
(3) To provide a means of communication among nurse anesthetists throughout the world
(4) To promote the independence of the nurse anesthetist as a professional specialist in nursing
(5) To advance the art and science of anesthesiology.[20]

This international organization of nurse specialists has the potential to be of great significance not only for nurse anesthetists, but for all of nursing. (One can only wonder what Dr. Frank McMechan would have made of this development.)

A third significant development occurring in 1978 was the founding of the first program offering a master's of science degree in nurse anesthesia. This was the result of the work of Joyce Kelly, CRNA, who affiliated the Kaiser Permanente Program with the Department of Nursing at California State University. Kelly received the first annual "Helen Lamb Outstanding Educator Award" in 1980. The following year this award was given to John Garde, CRNA, who implemented a master's program for CRNAs at Wayne State University in 1979.

The Road to Direct Reimbursement

In 1982 the Health Care Financing Administration (HCFA) proposed reimbursement regulations for anesthesiologists who direct or supervise CRNAs. The ASA had proposed that anesthesiologists not be allowed to be reimbursed for direction of more than two CRNAs, and the proposed regulation reflected this restrictive ratio. AANA's membership, along with some anesthesiologists (particularly from the Southeast), opposed this regulation, but stated that, if such a regulation were essential, a four-to-one ratio would be more in the public interest in terms of cost effectiveness. They based their argument on the fact that larger numbers of anesthesiologists would be more costly, and that those groups where there were higher ratios of CRNAs-to-anesthesiologists were more apt to accept Medicare assignments. This reasoning prevailed with HCFA in the final regulations.

Prospective payment legislation was passed by the US Congress in 1983, and was implemented in October of that year. This legislation inadvertently created reimbursement disincentives to the utilization of CRNAs, since CRNA services had to be reimbursed as a part of the DRG (Diagnostic Related Group), while anesthesiologist reimbursement was unaffected. Such an incentive made it possible for hospitals to eliminate their CRNA costs by terminating the employment of their CRNAs and shifting these services to anesthesiologists and their groups, thus reaping a "windfall" from the DRG. In addition, since the DRG was established on the basis of a pooled mean from hospitals that employed CRNAs and those that did not, the DRG would not, in any case, fully reimburse hospitals for their CRNA service. Thus, the PPS (Prospective Payment System), through its reimbursement incentives, did more to threaten the elimination or control of CRNAs than any other single incident in nurse anesthetist history.

This served as a basis for the AANA to seek regulatory or legislative relief from the HCFA and from the Congress. The Association did three things: (1) It requested a single exception to PPS from HCFA to allow anesthesiologists to charge for the services of CRNAs whom they employed under Part B of Medicare (this request was granted for a three-year period); (2) The AANA sought an amendment to the PPS legislation to provide a pass-through of reasonable CRNA costs to hospitals, which was in fact enacted in 1984, again for a three-year period; (3) The AANA, with Congressional assistance in both the House and Senate, had legislation introduced in both the 98th and 99th Congresses to amend the Social Security Act to provide for direct reimbursement legislation for the CRNAs. It took until October 21, 1986, for this to pass, but it was signed into law as of that date by President Ronald Reagan. Known as the Omnibus Budget Reconciliation Act of 1986 (OBRA), Section 9320 of the bill includes the AANA direct reimbursement package under Medicare for all CRNA services. This legislative passage and successive regulatory implementation phase pursued under the leadership of Association Presidents Patricia Fleming, CRNA, Patrick Downey, CRNA, Barbara Adams, CRNA, Richard Ouellette, CRNA, Peggy McFadden, CRNA, Mary Jeanette Mannino, CRNA, and Sandra M. Maree, CRNA, is considered to be one of the greatest lobbying achievements not only of the AANA, but of the whole of nursing.

The AANA's official position on the reimbursement issue has always been to avoid reimbursement disincentives pertaining to the utilization of CRNAs, as well as to promote healthy competition in the provision of anesthesia services. Furthermore, it has regarded anesthesiologist and CRNA services as requiring reimbursement from the same source, though not necessarily at the same scale.

In the final days before the implementation of direct reimbursement, the American Society of Anesthesiologists sought the support of the American Medical Association to oppose the proposed CRNA Medicare fee schedule. Despite this, implementation occurred on January 1, 1989. AANA President Sandra M. Maree, CRNA, noted that "Although some issues still need to be resolved, the 'bottom line' is that CRNAs now can be paid directly for their services under Medicare." She added, "Furthermore, we are the only nursing group to be accorded this distinction." Another note on the historical significance of the moment was sounded by the executive director of the American Nurses' Association. Dr. Judith A. Ryan said that "The American Association of Nurse Anesthetists' achievement to secure direct reimbursement for CRNAs is a singular, notable contribution to identification and payment of the nurse as a provider of care, and nursing services as covered health care benefits."[21]

"Plus Ça Change"

Also in 1983, following introduction of this important legislation, the ASA House of Delegates at its fall meeting passed a resolution that stated a regional anesthetic should be administered only by qualified physicians, despite disagreements with this action by a number of reputable anesthesiologists. Some of these others, however, upon returning to their places of practice, immediately issued policies precluding nurse anesthetists from providing regional anesthesia, as well as precluding teaching its administration in nurse anesthesia educational programs. The Maine Attorney General, as an example of the opposing view, was able to obtain a consent decree reversing this action in a hospital in Portland. However, this ASA resolution was followed by another one involving placement of intra-arterial lines. Where these two resolutions influenced departmental or hospital policy, the CRNA's practice has been significantly restricted. In addition to these, the ASA House of Delegates also passed another resolution precluding its members of the ASA-AANA Liaison Committee from meeting with AANA members until the AANA would accept the unilaterally developed Anesthesia Care Team statement, which was unacceptable to the AANA. As a result, no meetings of the liaison committee have since been held.

A worsening of the ASA-AANA tensions occurred during the years between 1983 and 1986, resulting from a variety of situations (not surprisingly, AANA President Patrick Downey initiated the "Dagmar Nelson Fund" during 1983–84 to help cover costs of legal challenges to nurse anesthetists). These situations included: projected overage of physicians and increase in the number of medical residents in anesthesiology, many at the expense of nurse anesthesia student spaces and of CRNAs, leading to the closure of numerous nurse anesthesia educational programs; an AANA brief in amicus curiae (written chiefly by Ira Gunn) to the US Supreme Court in the controversial Hyde Case, correcting the record pertaining to CRNAs reflected in the transcripts and court decisions at the lower court levels and also the Supreme Court's ruling against Hyde, which the ASA had supported in its own amicus curiae brief; the AANA legislative-regulatory activities at the national and selected state levels as they pertained to the Prospective Payment legislation, direct reimbursement, and clinical practice privileges; threats by some anesthesiologists of replacing CRNAs with physician assistants if the AANA persisted in this legislative lobbying program, particularly with regard to direct reimbursement, etc.

With soaring medical costs, shortages of hospital censuses, and the rise of Health Maintenance Organizations (HMOs), it seemed that anesthesiologists were fearful of losing their financial footing in the health care field to the advances of the nurse anesthetists. Hence, there was renewed conflict over money.

In another development of the 1983–85 period, liability insurance became an arena for increased pressure on nurse anesthetists. Surgeon's liability insurance coverages were increasingly threatened to be canceled, or additional premiums imposed if they continued to utilize CRNAs in their practice. The incidence of this activity appeared to occur chiefly in physician-owned insurance companies. Additional physician pressures were reported by Gunn:

> A variety of local problems have emerged following ASA meetings: anesthesiologists return to their practice area and take away selected employment benefits, such as payment of professional dues, and/or pressure their CRNA employees to write AANA telling them that they disagree with AANA's legislative program, etc. There have also been attempts to restrict nurse anesthetist practice through Medical Board or other non-Nursing Board regulations (Louisiana, New Jersey, Illinois, etc., or challenge state boards of nurse examiners by court suits pertaining to regulations issued concerning nurse anesthetists (Maryland, Texas).[22]

Powerful physician alliances also caused problems for nurse anesthetists. In particular, the physician-dominated Joint Commission on the Accreditation of Hospitals and the ASA set hospital standards which adversely impact CRNA practice and for which no validated studies exist to warrant such changes.[23] In formal responses to the JCAH, the AANA has continued to oppose such standards.

From Legality to Liability

The matter of the legality of nurse anesthetist practice was determined by the Dagmar Nelson case. The matter of liability of nurse anesthetists began being discussed with AANA members in 1948, when Association Counsel Emmanuel Hayt raised the question, "Do Anesthetists Need Liability Insurance?" The following year professional liability insurance was made available to the membership. It marked the beginning of the end for the concept of the surgeon as "Captain of the Ship."

There has been considerable controversy over the years regarding the liability of a surgeon for the negligent acts or omissions of persons giving him/her assistance with particular procedures. Because the legal concept of imputed negligence is in the process of evolution, there has been some confusion, not only among nurse anesthetists, but among other professionals as well. The general concept from which all other theories flow is the legal doctrine of *respondeat superior,* meaning that the negligent act of an employee will be imputed to the employer, even if the employer is not involved in the situation that caused an injury. This is based on the employer's technical right to select, train and control the acts of his/her employee.

One of the first expansions of this doctrine is the "borrowed servant doctrine," in which courts have decided that the services of an employee can be loaned to a third party for a temporary period of time and for the performance of specific tasks or functions. The loan of the employee includes a delegation of the right to direct or control his/her services to that third party. Thus, in imposing liability on a surgeon, the courts have stated that he/she is liable for the error of the temporary or borrowed servants (i.e., nurses). Courts have justified this position by stating that although employed by the hospital, nurses can become the temporary servants or agents of the attending surgeon during the course of an operation, and liability for their negligent acts may thus be imposed upon the surgeon under the doctrine of *respondeat superior.* However, in California, at least, this harsh application of doctrine has been abandoned.

Related to all of this is the doctrine of the "Captain of the Ship," in which (as in the navy), the courts hold the surgeon responsible for all the injuries that occur because of his/her status and presence in the operating room (as a captain is held responsible for the actions of his crew).

These legal theories have been utilized in courts of law to hold the physician liable for the negligence of others. Despite many cases in support of these kinds of imputed negligence, there appears to be a modern trend away from findings of vicarious liability simply because of a physician's status and presence during an operation. This new trend finds the surgeon liable only when he/she has participated in the negligent action. Courts in their jurisdictions have found neither a right nor a duty to control by surgeons.

The implications of this type of trend in liability cases support greater use of nurse anesthetists, nurses, and assistants in surgery. Since surgeons are less likely to be held responsible for the negligence of such personnel, one significant obstacle to employment of nurse anesthetists appears to have been removed (thwarting the aforementioned physician-owned insurance companies' attempts to keep them out by penalizing the premiums of surgeons who have used nurse anesthetists). This, however, does not reduce the threat of liability suits being directed at the nurse anesthetists individually, nor does it remove the need for liability insurance to protect themselves.

It does seem that the "Captain of the Ship" has departed from the legal battleground. The AANA's legal counsel, Gene A. Blumenreich, summarized the opposition argument as follows: "Because nurse anesthetists are medically directed by a physician, when surgeons work with nurse anesthetists the surgeons become liable for their mistakes—but when surgeons work with anesthesiologists, the surgeons do not have to worry about what happens at the head of the table."[24] Blumenreich argues that this position is groundless: "There are at least three things wrong with this premise. First, surgeons are not always liable for the negligence of nurse anesthetists. Second, surgeons may also be liable for the negligence of anesthesiologists. Third, because a surgeon's liability, whether working with nurse anesthetists or anesthesiologists, depends on the particular facts of the situation, as a practical matter, the surgeon is likely to be included in the suit whether the surgeon is working with a nurse anesthetist or an anesthesiologist."[25] Furthermore, he concludes that there has never been found a case (that is, an appellate decision) in which the surgeon was actually found liable for negligence of a nurse anesthetist based on the statutory obligation of supervision.

Blumenreich's argument continues, "The problem is that a surgeon's liability depends not on law, but on the facts. Did the surgeon do something wrong? Was the surgeon, in fact, in control? Courts will grant motions for summary judgment only if it is clear that there are no factual circumstances claimed under which the surgeon could be held liable. . . . Because the surgeon's liability for the negligence of a nurse anesthetist or an anesthesiologist depends on the specific facts of the case, it will be difficult in most cases for a court to grant summary judgment in favor of the surgeon." But as another practical matter, he also indicated, in liability or malpractice suits of this nature, everyone who has stood around the table—and then some—will as a matter of fact be entered as defendants in the suit. It may be found that all have been negligent by a jury, which then awards damages to a plaintiff that come from every defendant involved—and that is why nurse anesthetists need to have adequate professional liability coverage, and this is why the legal doctrine of "Captain of the Ship" no longer holds water.

The Hyde Case

Another legal problem that arose in the 1980s has been the determinations of hospitals to grant exclusive contracts to physicians or groups of physicians organized as a partnership or corporation to perform certain patient services, such as, for example, anesthesiologist groups that have exclusivity to practice in certain hospitals. But these groups may also employ nurse anesthetists themselves (this situation may bring to mind the much earlier statement by Dr.Ralph Waters, criticizing the doctor who wanted his office girl to administer anesthetics because she worked so cheaply). So, where such arrangements are granted in anesthesiology departments, nurse anesthetists are likely to find themselves on all sides of the issue. If, however, the hospital's arrangements preclude them from rendering services at that hospital, the nurse anesthetists are then in the same position as a physician who has been excluded from serving patients at that hospital. Other possibilities in these cases include: the nurse benefits by being employed by the anesthesiologist group granted the exclusive privilege, or the nurse anesthetists may even continue to be employed by the hospital and remain unaffected by any contract with third-party outside practitioners.

There can be little wonder that these kinds of complex situations end up in court.

The case of *Hyde v. E. Jefferson Parish Hospital District No. 2* is such a one. Here the Louisiana court refused to find that the hospital's arrangement with a group to provide anesthesia services was in violation of antitrust laws or of equal protection or due process. These theories had been advanced by a nongroup anesthesiologist who had been denied appointment to the medical staff by virtue of the exclusive arrangement. Instead, the court adopted the hospital's rationale in contracting for exclusive anesthesia services. The hospital contended, among other things, that the system facilitated the scheduling of surgeries, gave a more efficient use of operating rooms, permitted the hospital governing board to monitor more closely the professional standards used by the members of this group, and ensured the availability of anesthesia services to hospital patients.

But this matter was not resolved. Dr. Edwin Hyde appealed, and the Fifth Circuit Court of Appeals reversed the trial court's decision. The higher court disagreed with the trial court as to the market area of East Jefferson Hospital, finding that it was much smaller than the trial court had found. The appellate court held that the arrangement between the hospital and Dr. Hyde was illegal under the antitrust laws by its mere existence. In addition, the Court of Appeals discussed a number of anticompetitive effects that such an exclusive contract engendered.

Under the surface were the court's attempts to understand and describe any relevant economics. The economics in this case clearly involved nurse anesthetists, since one of the justifications given by the hospital for entering into the exclusive contract was that it permitted greater use of CRNAs. The appellate court therefore saw the role of

CRNAs as a crucial issue: "Another twist which is important to an understanding of the specialty [anesthesiology] is that more than in any other specialty, anesthesiology had been confronted with the growth of a paraprofessional counterpart—the anesthetist. Herein lies the actual basis for the hospital's actions in this case."[26]

But this was not the end of it. The hospital requested that the US Supreme Court hear the case. Because of the lower courts' discussions of the CRNAs, and because the legal status of exclusive contracts between hospitals and anesthesiologists is obviously of importance to the AANA and its members, the AANA decided to file an amicus curiae brief with the Supreme Court. The complexity of the situation for the AANA stemmed from the fact that the interests of CRNAs are varied. While many CRNAs are employed by hospitals that have exclusive contracts with anesthesiologists and might be adversely affected by "open" staff, other CRNAs have brought their own lawsuits similar to that of Dr. Hyde. Therefore, the AANA Board of Directors determined that the Association would neither support nor oppose exclusive contracts. Rather, the board decided to file the brief in order to correct the impression of the role of CRNAs which had emerged from the language of the District and Appellate Courts' opinions.

The US Supreme Court heard the Hyde case, and on March 26, 1984, issued its decision upholding the legality of an exclusive contract between a hospital and a group of anesthesiologists.

This decision is of interest to nurse anesthetists because the court did, in fact, refrain from making deprecating remarks regarding nurse anesthetists, and because of the reasoning upholding the legality of exclusive contracts. Its decision was written by Justice Stevens, who was joined by Justices Brennan, Marshall, White, and Blackmun. A separate opinion, agreeing with the result but not with the reasoning, was written by Justice O'Connor and joined in by Chief Justice Burger, and Justices Powell and Rhenquist (hence, the decision was actually unanimous). The significance of the two "reasoning" opinions is that, although they both agreed that the contract did not violate antitrust laws, the opinions approached the matter in different ways. Also, in this case, the majority opinion was separated by a single vote from the concurring opinion. Therefore, Justice O'Connor's reasoning is not the official reasoning of the court, because the majority opinion was the opinion of the more senior members of the court, but the concurring opinion may be the way the Supreme Court will approach these cases in the future, as the personnel of the court continues to change. Her opinion requires a weighing of the benefits and detriments of each anticompetitive arrangement, an analysis she claimed was engaged in, in fact, under all per se cases. Justice O'Connor would eliminate the entire concept of the per se rule. She wrote:

"The time has therefore come to abandon the *'per se'* label and refocus the inquiry on the adverse economic effects, and the potential economic benefits, that the tie may have."[27] She further suggested a test for analyzing the exclusive contract, and concluded that there is no good economic reason for treating surgery and anesthesia as if they were separate services. According to Justice O'Connor, the arrangements offered by an exclusive contract actually improve patient care and allow the hospital to operate more efficiently, which is what the Jefferson Hospital attorneys had argued all along.

On October 2, 1985, the United States Court of Appeals for the Ninth Circuit ruled in the case of *Bhan v. NME Hospitals, Inc.,* that nurse anesthetists have standing to sue under federal antitrust law for anticompetitive practices excluding them from the market for anesthesia services. The principle was established that CRNAs compete with anesthesiologists in providing services to hospitals, patients, and other doctors, and that anticompetitive arrangements designed to exclude CRNAs from practice may be challenged under the antitrust laws. The court said: "A nurse anesthetist administering anesthesia under the supervision of a physician may still duplicate many of the services provided by an M.D. anesthesiologist."

The principle established in the Bhan case was applied a year later when a nurse anesthetist was awarded substantial damages in an antitrust case brought against a hospital and a group of anesthesiologists. In *Oltz v. St. Peter's Community Hospital,* a federal jury in Montana awarded damages to a CRNA, finding that he was the victim of an exclusive contract between an anesthesia group run by four anesthesiologists and a Helena hospital—a contract that illegally discriminated against him.

With the increasing number of physicians, decreasing number of nurses, slowing economic growth, and consumer resistance to higher health-care costs, the kinds of competitive conflicts discussed above seem likely to remain with nurse anesthetists. It is not surprising, then, that the 1989 president of the American Association of Nurse Anesthetists, Sandra Maree, chose for the theme of her tenure, "Strength in Unity." In her inaugural address she reminded some 23,000 members that, while nurse anesthetist diversity in practice settings, education, personal and professional interests, and goals must continue to be respected, unity remained the key to their future:

Although individuality, creativity, and freedom are essential to human progress and professional growth, the interdependence of health providers and complexity of issues that must be faced today prohibit complete professional freedom. The health-care system of today is in major transition, and change will occur with/or without our involvement. If we are to remain a viable provider in the system, our major goals and focus must be compatible with the needs of society. We must study the issues, seek the assistance of experts when necessary, and speak with one voice on those major issues which will determine our right to practice and educate our successors. Our greatest strength has been that this organization speaks for 97 percent of all CRNAs in this country—a group which directly administers well over 50 percent of all anesthetics in this country, and about 70 percent of those in rural communities. With one voice, we have and are addressing the major issues regarding our right to practice; this must not change in the future.

Our profession today is like a river with streams branching off along the way. As individuals, we are like tiny rafts with little or no power to overcome the currents. We constantly pass opportunities to take a different channel, and without a view of the entire river, we may take the wrong course. If we make no choice, time and the river will make it for us. The key to controlling our destiny is to make choices together that chart our course, and to pull on those oars in unison to arrive at our chosen destination.

The entire history of the nurse anesthetist experience bears witness to the wisdom of her words.

Appendix I

Past Presidents
of the
American Association of Nurse Anesthetists

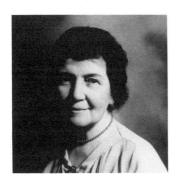

1931–33   Agatha C. Hodgins

"From whatever angle the subject is considered, the school remains the repository of our hopes, the guarantee of security for our association."

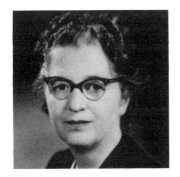

1933–35   Gertrude Fife

"The formation of this organization was for the purpose of elevating the standard of anesthesia."

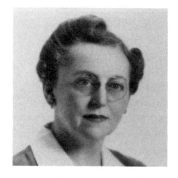

1935–37   Hilda Salomon

"During the term of my office a sincere effort has been made not only to continue along the line of the outstanding achievements of the past, but in addition looking to the future to nurture and increase the value and importance of this national organization throughout the country."

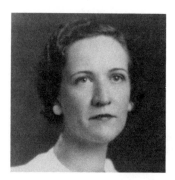

1937–40   Miriam Shupp

"We are living in the midst of troubled and doubtful times, and we know not what the future holds for us either as individuals or as an organization, but let us pursue our course, as individuals and as an organization, following the belief of that wise philosopher, Ralph Waldo Emerson, who said, 'Work and learn—there is but only one liberator in this life, and that is Endeavor, earnest, entire, perennial Endeavor.'"

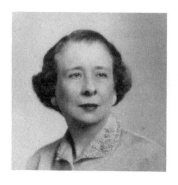

1940–42   Helen Lamb Powell Frost

"The history of our Association from its inception has been one of constructive onward and upward progress, surmounting obstacles as they arose, driving ever forward to higher levels of accomplishment and ideals of service."

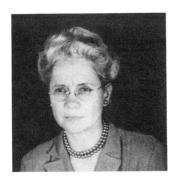

1942–44   Rosalie McDonald

"Each member must realize that cooperation and activity are essential in making the state associations a bulwark upon which the national organization may draw when the need arises. Our national strength and growth rest upon the state and sectional associations."

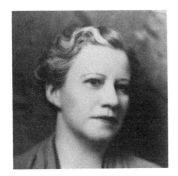

1944–46   Hazel Blanchard

"The objects of this Association are: to advance the science and art of anesthesiology, to develop educational standards, to facilitate cooperation between nurse anesthetists, hospitals and the medical profession, to publish bulletins, to maintain a central office for information and reference and to promulgate an educational program. These objectives do not change and should be constantly kept in mind."

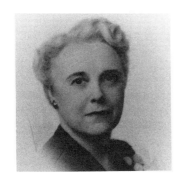

1946–48   Lucy Richards

"As individuals and as an association, we must find means of cooperating with nurses, individually and through their associations, with physicians, individually and through their associations, and with hospital administrators, individually and through their associations. When the day comes that our successors can add the realization of that objective to the past accomplishments of nurse anesthetists and the Association, then we shall truly have come of age."

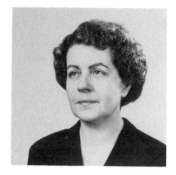

1948–50   Myra Van Arsdale

"Our greatest responsibility is toward our educational objectives."

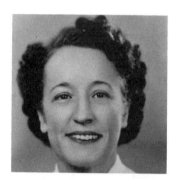

1950–52   Verna Bean

"It is my happy duty to tell you that your dream has come true, and that formal accreditation of schools has become an actuality."

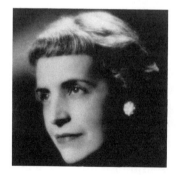

1952–54   Josephine Bunch

"We realize that we have gone far in our efforts to improve the quality of anesthesia service. We realize that we are doing many things that have been but dreams in the not too distant past. We acknowledge our great debt to those who plan before our ideals are reached. We know that we have the strength of high purpose. We ask for the wisdom to achieve greater things for the good of mankind."

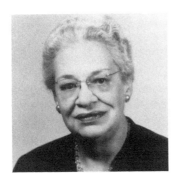

1954–56   Minnie Haas

"I believe that I will serve you better if I offer to you a suggestion for the future: Do not be discouraged by this period of unrest."

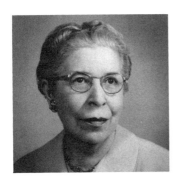

1956–58   Lillian Baird

"We must watch for every opportunity to raise the standard of service and to conform to the high ethical principles that have been adopted by this Association."

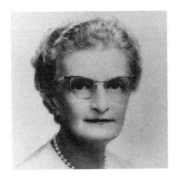

1958–60   Olive Berger

"If you believe that many members working together can accomplish more than individuals working alone, we will find the enthusiasm necessary for group action."

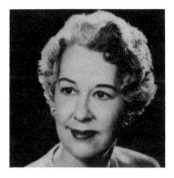

1960–61   Evelyn Auld

"You have confirmed my belief that so long as we keep our standards high and so long as we continue to give the good service to which we are dedicated, our future will be secure."

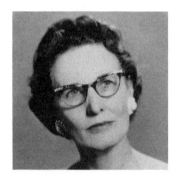

1961–62   Jessie Compton

"It is our belief that professional associations such as ours must work toward the ideals for which we aspire. We must constantly strive to improve the service which is the basis for our entire existence. We believe that those of us who work in this profession should constantly strive to improve the qualifications in order that we will be able to command, not to demand, the recognition and remunerations to which we are entitled."

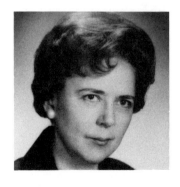

1962–63   Martha Belew

"Each year we are privileged to carry the programs forward a little further toward our goals. It is only by the cooperative efforts of many persons that we are able to progress."

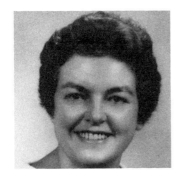

1963–64   Mary Alice Costello

"I have learned that we cannot walk alone toward our goals."

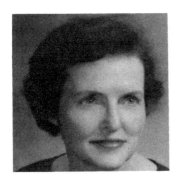

1964–65   Mabel Courtney

"So long as we continue to select our leaders wisely and so long as we support them diligently, we may assure ourselves that our Association will continue to grow, and grow not only in membership, but in professional stature."

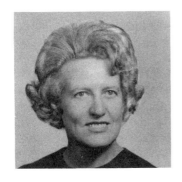

1965–66   Helen Vos

"This is our 35th year. We owe the founders of the American Association of Nurse Anesthetists a word of thanks. Some are with us today and, speaking for the entire membership, to all those who gave us a good beginning we express our gratitude for your efforts and sacrifices."

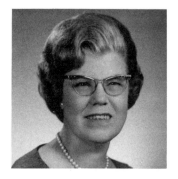

1966–67   Hazel Currier

"I believe that there is no limit to the good that the Association can do if its members continue to subscribe to the thesis that security for the individual member is not a primary goal and that united action by our highly-motivated professional people can be, as it has been for me, a most rewarding experience."

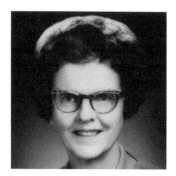

1967–68   Rose Featherston

"It has been a pleasure working with the Board of Trustees, with the Committees and with the members of the Executive Staff. Without their loyalty and support no progress could have been made by one member such as I, even with the distinguished title of President."

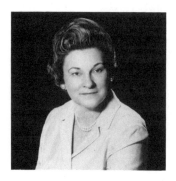

1968–69   Marie N. Bader

"We have been a vigorous organization. We have tried to remain within a realistic pattern of goals. We believe that if the members will continue to rise to the challenge that is placed before them, not only by their fellow members but by society as a whole, we will be able to make even greater progress in the future."

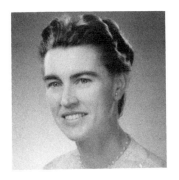

1969–70   Virginia Gaffey

"This year saw the end of an era. Miss Florence McQuillen has worked tirelessly, diligently, conscientiously, and patiently for the cause of the AANA. Seven days a week, as many hours as needed in a day, she has labored since 1948 in our behalf. For myself, and on behalf of the entire membership, I would like to thank her for her hours of devotion and work. Miss McQuillen, you and our leaders of the past have built our Association to the esteem that we now enjoy. I trust that our future leaders and members will maintain the high standards which have been set for AANA."

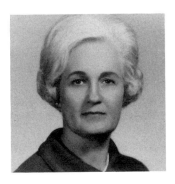

1970–71   Vella G. Nelson

"The professional responsibilities and the stature of the Certified Registered Nurse Anesthetist have never been greater; however, the stature of the CRNA will increase with continuing education."

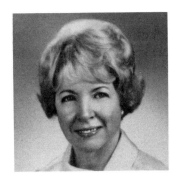

1971–72   Carol Abbey

"In the past, strength of unity and team action have guided us. The future continued high standards through performance and discipline will also guide us. As we grow in numbers, may we mature even more in self-respect and public esteem. We must continue to earn the reputation of achievement through professional excellence and humanism by individual members and the American Association of Nurse Anesthetists."

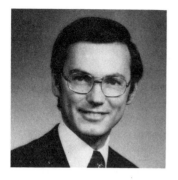

1972–73   John F. Garde

"Growth of the AANA has been an integral part of the growth and virtual transformation of the entire health field, now facing such complicated social and economic factors as the increase in size and mobility of population, the urbanization of society and the public concern for health delivery."

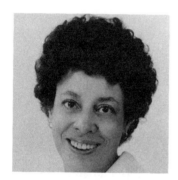

1973–74   Goldie D. Brangman

"An effective organization continually looks for ways to involve members in the development of plans, policies, and procedures on a year-round basis, because through participation comes understanding, and members can then, as a rule, wholeheartedly support the interim decisions and actions of their Board."

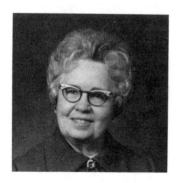

1974–75   Mildred Rumpf

"Ships do not drift into ports; they are steered in by experts. Individual people are the doers. There are no magic shortcuts, and survival is dependent upon one's ability to meet challenges."

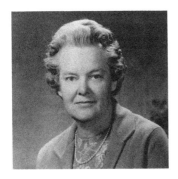

1975–76   Dolores Biggins

"The professional goals set down by the founders of this organization were achieved by human beings like ourselves. Their efforts and sacrifices made possible the AANA of today; and by helping put the present in perspective with the past, the AANA can prepare for the future with more confidence."

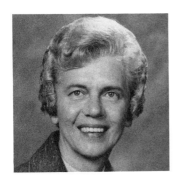

1976–77   Ruth Ecklund

"With the foresight and determination of our founders and our predecessors, we continue to be a viable association. We are continually reminded of our objectives and the need to explore ways in which they can be best achieved for the good of each member. Periodically, it becomes necessary to review and update such objectives to meet current concerns. Traditionalism is fine in part; however, it must give way to present and future needs."

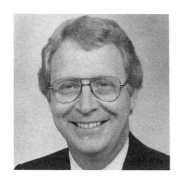

1977–78   Ronald F. Caulk

"Our first leaders set for us a strong foundation on which we have expanded and grown. We will continue to grow as our Founders did, with the spirit of adventure and with unity and accountability."

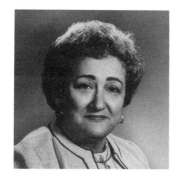

1978–79   Josephine A. Nickel

"A great debt of gratitude is due to each and every Committee of this organization. Their members—all volunteers—have worked long and diligently on their assignments and have performed well."

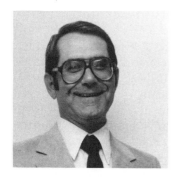

1979–80   Jimmy N. Kerley

"As we approach the Golden Anniversary year of our Association let us all be mindful that it was no small effort for us to attain the professional stature we have today; and for tomorrow, though the work will be as demanding, we can accomplish much through a united effort."

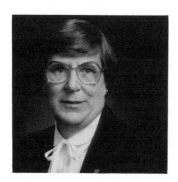

1980–81   Kathryn L. Wagner

"Our educators are the initial providers of anesthesia personnel and should be recognized as such. Young anesthetists should be encouraged along the educator career path as well."

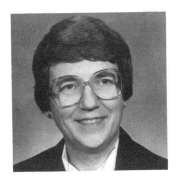

1981–82 Sandra J. Kilde

"In the 50-year history of our Association, we have accomplished high standards and excellence in the care of our patients, in the education of our nurse anesthesia students and in the continuing education provided to our certified members. Other nursing associations look to the AANA and its many accomplishments. They perceive the AANA as a role model in developing many of their own programs."

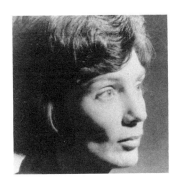

1982–83 Patricia R. Fleming

"I believe it is time that we recognize: that differences of opinion provide the best debates; that decision making achieves its highest potential when we have several options from which to choose; and that consensus, rather than confrontation, has the most potential for building a future with which we can all live. Consensus can only come through negotiations of positions and negotiation depends upon an openness and a willingness to bring members of varying opinions into our deliberations."

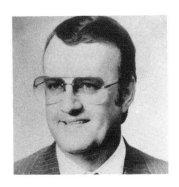

1983–84 Patrick M. Downey

"There will certainly continue to be threats to our existence and to our practice—but we must recognize that that has been the history of this profession. It has also been the reason we have survived and thrived. We have been made strong by the fires of adversity instead of allowing them to consume us. We have come through with sharper edges and brighter visions."

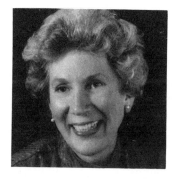

1984–85   Barbara V. Adams

"Our Association is one of the leading organizations in nursing today. The reason for our leadership and our strength is our unity of purpose and dedication to our profession. One of the responsibilities of a profession is to make advances in research and to inform the public as to its advances. We can increase our strength, and we can advance our profession, by promoting our Educational and Research Foundation."

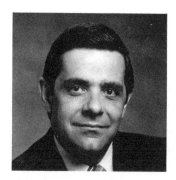

1985–86   Richard G. Ouellette

"We go forward today as an Association still strong in its youth and powerful in its purpose. With our spirit renewed, and with our commitment to the public we serve intact, with our alliances strengthened, with our influential and political endeavors placing us in a leadership position in this age of health care, we look to a future rich in possibilities. All of this because we worked and acted together, not as individuals, but collectively as an Association."

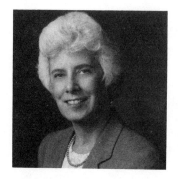

1986–87   Peggy L. McFadden

"I am grateful to those people who have brought us to this place in history—and they are many—but, I believe the past is to be learned from, not to live in, so we must move forward. We cannot be so gratified in our accomplishments that we fail to recognize the need to set new goals and to make new challenges instead of reacting to those designed by others. Indeed, I believe, we should be part of *creating* the future."

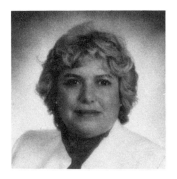

1987–88   Mary Jeanette Mannino

"The American Association of Nurse Anesthetists has a remarkable history and will continue to be a compelling force in health care in the present and the future. From the pioneers of our profession, through the participation of nurse anesthetists in the major military conflicts, to the progressive sophisticated practitioners, CRNAs provide quality anesthesia care with dedication, skill, and commitment."

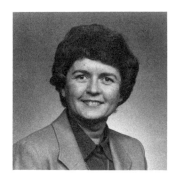

1988–89   Sandra M. Maree

"Our greatest strength has been that this organization speaks for 97 percent of all CRNAs in this country—a group which directly administers well over 50 percent of all anesthetics in this country, and about 70 percent of those in rural communities. *With one voice, we have and are addressing the major issues regarding our right to practice; this must not change in the future.*"

Appendix II

**Current Requirements for a Career as a
Certified Registered Nurse Anesthetist**

- A Bachelor of Science in Nursing (B.S.N.) or other appropriate baccalaureate degree.
- A current R.N. license.
- At least one year of experience in an acute care nursing setting.
- A minimum of two years of education beyond nursing school in an accredited program of nurse anesthesia, *including a clinical practicum in a university-based or large community hospital.* (The majority of programs offer a master's degree to those who have completed the nurse anesthesia curriculum.)
- The successful completion of a national certification examination.
- The successful completion of a continuing education and recertification program every two years.

Appendix III

Recipients of "Awards of Appreciation"

1947 Barnes Hospital
1948 Dr. George W. Crile, MD (posthumously)
1950 Gertrude L. Fife
1951 Mae B. Cameron
1953 Agnes McGee
1954 Hospital Sisters of the Third Order of St. Francis, Springfield, Illinois
1956 Helen Lamb and Lucy Richards
1958 Hilda Salomon
1959 Verna Rice

Honorary Membership (Non-Anesthetist)

1960 Cameron W. Meredith
1984 Betty A. Colitti

Special Recognition Award

1988 John R. Mannix

Appendix IV

Recipients of "The Agatha Hodgins Award for Outstanding Accomplishment"

The Agatha Hodgins Award for Outstanding Accomplishment was established in 1975 to recognize individuals whose foremost dedication to excellence has furthered the art and science of nurse anesthesia.

The award was established in honor of Agatha Hodgins (1877–1945), founder and first president of the American Association of Nurse Anesthetists. Miss Hodgins was one of the first to perfect the nitrous oxide–oxygen technique of anesthesia, and was instrumental in establishing nurse anesthesia as a profession.

1975   Ruth P. Satterfield

Miss Satterfield, honored for her contributions to nurse anesthesia education, spent the majority of her career in the United States Army. She opened an anesthesia course at Fort Jackson, North Carolina, in 1941. Then, in the early fifties, she developed one of the first educationally structured nurse anesthesia programs for the army. She was the first recipient of the army's "A" prefix for professional excellence, an award equal to academic professorial rank. Miss Satterfield was the first *nurse* ever to be appointed consultant to the Army Surgeon General, and was the first person to assume responsibility for directing all army nurse anesthesia programs. Following her retirement from the army in 1968, Miss Satterfield has served as an Education Consultant to the AANA and the Council on Accreditation.

1976   Helen Lamb

One of the founding members of the AANA, Helen Lamb was truly a pioneer in the field of anesthesia. She founded the School of Anesthesia at Barnes Hospital in St. Louis, Missouri, in 1929. She collaborated with Dr. Richard von Foregger in the development of the von Foregger anesthesia machine, and she performed the anesthetic for the world's first successful pneumonectomy as anesthetist for Dr. Evarts Graham. Mrs. Lamb contributed a chapter on endotracheal anesthesia to Dr. Graham's book, *Thoracic Surgery,* which has become a classic. She served as chairman of the Education Committee from 1931 to 1939, and established the curriculum and minimum standards for schools of nurse anesthesia. She was AANA president in 1940–42.

1977   Hilda Salomon

Miss Salomon, a charter member of the AANA, began her anesthesia career in 1922 at the Jewish Hospital in Philadelphia, where she later became director of the School of Anesthesia. During her many years of participation in the AANA, her farsighted leadership was evident many times over. In fact, during her two years as president of the Association in 1935–37, she was considered too radical by some when she proposed that the membership be opened to include men and black nurse anesthetists, a step that finally occurred as a result of the crisis of World War II.

1978   Gertrude Fife

Mrs. Fife was Agatha Hodgins's first assistant at the Lakeside School of Anesthesia at the time of the organizational meeting; it was she who made the motion to form the Association at that meeting. When Agatha Hodgins became ill in 1933, Mrs. Fife assumed Miss Hodgins's administrative roles in both the AANA and at Lakeside Hospital. She coordinated the first Annual Meeting in 1933, held in Milwaukee, and was elected president at that meeting. Mrs. Fife was the first editor of the AANA's official publication, the *Bulletin,* serving in that position from 1933–45. She was AANA treasurer from 1935 to 1950, and was a staunch advocate of the accreditation process for schools. With Helen Lamb and Miriam Shupp, she developed the mechanics for the Qualifying Examination, first given in 1945.

1979   Helen Vos

Miss Vos was directly responsible for the education of countless numbers of nurse anesthesia students now practicing throughout the country and across the globe. She was education director of the Barnes Hospital Anesthesia School in St. Louis, and served as director of the anesthesia program at Hurley Hospital in Flint, Michigan; United Christian Hospital in Lahore, Pakistan; and North Carolina Baptist Hospital in Winston-Salem, North Carolina, where she was also appointed Assistant Professor of the Bowman Gray School of Medicine. She served as AANA president from 1965–66, and also served on the Council on Practice of Nurse Anesthesia.

1980   Olive Berger

Miss Berger completed her anesthesia training in 1922 at Johns Hopkins Hospital in Baltimore, Maryland. In 1931, she was named chief anesthetist there, a position she held until her retirement in 1967. As chief anesthetist, she managed the anesthesia department, administered anesthesia, and trained at least four nurse anesthesia students a year. She administered the anesthesia for the first total pneumonectomy performed at Johns Hopkins and, with Helen Lamb, developed an endotracheal technique for intrathoracic surgery. She was the first nurse anesthetist to administer anesthesia to infants for repair of tetralogy of Fallot. She served as AANA president in 1958–60.

1981   Florence A. McQuillen

Florence McQuillen began her anesthesia career in 1927 when she joined the staff of the Mayo Clinic in Rochester, Minnesota, at the invitation of Dr. John Lundy. She began abstracting articles for publication in *Anesthesia Abstracts,* compiled by the Journal Club of the Mayo Clinic, and quickly assumed sole responsibility for the entire enterprise; she continued this solo effort until 1965. She also served on the AANA Public Relations Committee and as associate editor. From 1948–70, Miss McQuillen served as executive director of the AANA, and was influential in its growth and expansion in a variety of areas. In 1948, AANA membership numbered 3,200 nurse anesthetists; at the end of 1970, this number swelled to 14,500. Miss McQuillen was instrumental in gaining recognition for the AANA from such external organizations as the American Hospital Association and the US Department of Health, Education and Welfare (HEW) for its functions of accreditation and certification.

1982   Sister Yvonne Jenn

A nationally known educator of nurse anesthetists, Sister Yvonne founded the St. Francis School of Anesthesia in LaCrosse, Wisconsin, in 1942, and served as its director until her retirement in 1981. According to Dr. David Rho, director of the anesthesiology department at St. Francis Medical Center, "While Sr. Yvonne limited her time to one geographical city, touching lives directly in this community, she has produced hundreds of well qualified nurse anesthetists who are now, generations and life-times away, scattered throughout the United States and the world in such places as Japan, Korea, and Guatemala. Sr. Yvonne, through her graduates, is changing for the better hundreds of thousands of lives throughout the world." In addition to her role as educator of nurse anesthetists, Sr. Yvonne was a pioneer in the field of respiratory therapy, becoming one of the first Registered Respiratory Therapists in this country. She also served as president of the Wisconsin Association of Nurse Anesthetists.

1983   Ira P. Gunn

Miss Gunn distinguished herself in many areas relating to nurse anesthesia, including practice, research, education, publications, consultation, credentialing, and government relations. In 1968 she developed the first academic graduate program for nurse anesthetists, a joint venture between the US Army and the University of Hawaii. She spent twenty-one years in the US Army, serving as director of Army Nurse Anesthesiology courses at Tripler Army Medical Center in Hawaii, and at Walter Reed Army Medical Center in Washington, DC. She retired with numerous honors, including appointment as Consultant to the Army Surgeon General for Anesthesiology Nursing. She later served as visiting professor and director of the Nurse Anesthesia Program at State University of New York in Buffalo and Buffalo Veterans Administration Medical Center. Miss Gunn was the architect of the Council structure within the AANA, and served as project director for the Council on Accreditation petitions to the US Office of Education in 1975, 1976, and 1979. In 1981 she was elected a Fellow in the American Academy of Nursing. Miss Gunn contributed monumentally to the amicus curiae brief presented to the US Supreme Court by the AANA in regard to the Hyde case.

1984   Sophie Gran Winton

A practicing nurse anesthetist for more than fifty years, Mrs. Winton was given the Agatha Hodgins Award at the age of ninety-seven. She was a nurse anesthesia pioneer who provided financial support for the Dagmar Nelson trial in California, a test case that established the legal right of trained nurse anesthetists to their practice. She served as a nurse anesthetist during World War I in the American Expeditionary Forces in France, and was awarded the Croix de Guerre, as well as six overseas bars. She began her anesthesia career in 1913, working at Swedish Hospital in Minneapolis, and also worked for J. A. Heidbrink, demonstrating his anesthetic equipment. During the 1940s, she opened an out-patient plastic surgery clinic in Hollywood, numbering among her patients many film stars of the era.

1984   Miriam Shupp

A charter member of the AANA, Miss Shupp served as the Association's president from 1937–40. She was the only person to hold that office for three terms. For more than thirty-eight years, she was active in both clinical and educational endeavors. She was instrumental in developing anesthesia certification of nurse anesthetists, and chaired a committee that implemented the certifying examination. Miss Shupp published a number of papers on education and clinical subjects, and was thought to be the first to publish a report on controlled respiration with an anesthesia ventilator. In 1946 she succeeded Gertrude Fife as director of the School of Anesthesia at University Hospitals of Cleveland. She moved to Arizona in 1953, working as the sole anesthetist in a copper mining town.

1985   Del Portzer

In her twenty years as a clinician, instructor, and researcher at the Cleveland Clinic, Del Portzer was known for her research efforts in tandem with surgeons and anesthesiologists who pioneered much of modern surgical and anesthetic techniques. She served as director of the Cleveland Clinic School of Anesthesia from 1969 to 1973. She later worked as a staff nurse anesthetist at AMI Palm Beach Gardens Medical Center in Palm Beach Gardens, Florida. She developed a monograph that was adopted as a procedural manual for the department of anesthesia at St. Mary's Hospital in West Palm Beach, Florida, where she served as chief nurse anesthetist. Mrs. Portzer was particularly knowledgeable in cardiac anesthesia, and contributed to a book on coronary artery disease written by a physician colleague. She was a member of the Council on Nurse Anesthesia Practice, assisting in the drafting of the Standards of Practice. She served on the Advisory Board of *Current Reviews for Nurse Anesthetists.*

1986   Jessie Compton

Mrs. Compton's anesthesia career had a span of nearly fifty years, twenty-five of which she spent as department head and chief anesthetist at Methodist Hospital in Dallas. For eighteen years, she was department head and chief anesthetist at Chester Clinic and Hospital. She was a 1938 graduate of Baylor School of Anesthesia. In 1961–62 she served as AANA president, presiding over an administration that emphasized the importance of communicating the role of nurse anesthetist to the public. She served on many AANA committees, including the Public Relations Committee and Government Relations Committee, and was also president of the Texas Association of Nurse Anesthetists.

1987   Patricia Fleming

Mrs. Fleming was the first chairman of the Council on Certification of Nurse Anesthetists, and played a large role in the Council's initial development. In 1982–83 she served as president of the AANA. She remained active in government affairs for the Association, serving as Government Relations Committee chairman in 1984. Mrs. Fleming was a member of the editorial board of *CRNA Forum*. She was educated in anesthesia at Charity Hospital School of Nurse Anesthesia in New Orleans, and served for many years as chief nurse anesthetist at Wesley Long Community Hospital in Greensboro, North Carolina.

1988   Martha J. Lundgaard

Mrs. Lundgaard, a pioneer in health care and anesthesia in Minnesota, graduated from the Nurse Anesthesia Program at the University of Minnesota in 1934, following her training at the Lutheran Deaconess Hospital School of Nursing. After serving as supervisor of the Nurse Anesthesia Program at Minneapolis General Hospital, Mrs. Lundgaard held the position of consultant in nurse anesthesia for the Minnesota Department of Health from 1956 to 1974, where among her many activities, she assessed anesthesia services, developed a nurse anesthetist recruitment program, and conducted 765 training programs in cardiopulmonary resuscitation. Mrs. Lundgaard served on the AANA Examination Committee from 1945 to 1951 and as president of the Minnesota Association of Nurse Anesthetists in the mid-fifties. She conducted continuing education workshops through the University of Minnesota for twenty years and regional anesthesia refresher courses for ten years, and even found time to complete her baccalaureate degree in 1976. She retired in 1982.

Appendix V

Recipients of "The Helen Lamb Outstanding Educator Award"

The Helen Lamb Outstanding Educator Award is presented to a CRNA who has made a significant contribution to the education of nurse anesthetists. The award recognizes the individual's commitment to the profession of nurse anesthesia and to the advancement of educational standards that further the art and science of anesthesiology and result in high quality patient care.

The award was established in honor of Helen Lamb (1900–1979), founder and director of Barnes Hospital School of Anesthesia in St. Louis from 1929 to 1951. As chairman of the AANA Education Committee from 1931 through 1939, she established the curriculum and minimum standards for schools of nurse anesthesia. She pioneered endotracheal techniques in lung surgery and performed the anesthetic for the world's first successful pneumonectomy as anesthetist for the eminent surgeon, Dr. Evarts Graham. Helen Lamb served as president of the AANA from 1940 to 1942.

1980   Joyce Kelly

An active participant in the voluntary continuing education program of the AANA, Mrs. Kelly in 1971 conducted a study on the feasibility of developing a nurse anesthesia program for Kaiser Permanente Hospital in Los Angeles. Due to her efforts, the school was formed, and Mrs. Kelly was named director. In 1978 she worked to affiliate the Kaiser Permanente program with the Department of Nursing at California State University, thereby founding the first program offering a master of science degree in nurse anesthesia. She lectures widely on clinical anesthesia and has written and produced a number of educational films about anesthesia administration. Mrs. Kelly has been a member of the *AANA Journal* Editorial Advisory Board. She served on the AANA Board of Directors as a regional director, and was then elected to the offices of AANA treasurer and vice president.

1981   John F. Garde

Prior to becoming AANA education director in September, 1980, Mr. Garde was associate professor and chairman of the Department of Anesthesia, College of Pharmacy and Allied Health Professions, Wayne State University, a position he assumed in 1972 when the university implemented the baccalaureate degree program for nurse anesthetists. He implemented the master's program for CRNAs in 1979. He was also program director for the Program of Nurse Anesthesia at Wayne State University from 1964–72. He served as chief nurse anesthetist at Detroit General Hospital for more than fifteen years, from 1964 to 1980. Mr. Garde has served on numerous AANA committees. He chaired the Education Committee in 1967–68 and again from 1974–76. He became a member of the Board in 1968 and served as trustee, vice president and president-elect. He was elected president of the AANA in 1972, becoming the first male (and youngest) CRNA to hold that position. A graduate of the Alexian Brothers Hospital School of Nursing in Chicago, Illinois, he completed his anesthesia education at St. Francis Hospital School of Anesthesia in LaCrosse, Wisconsin. He received his Bachelor's degree in Psychology from the University of Detroit and earned his master's degree in physiology from Wayne State University in Detroit, Michigan.

1982   Virginia A. Gaffey

Miss Gaffey rendered years of service on behalf of nurse anesthesia education as an on-site visitor for the Council on Accreditation of Nurse Anesthesia Educational Programs/Schools, and as a member of the Council on Certification of Nurse Anesthetists. She contributed several articles to the *AANA Journal* during her career. Miss Gaffey was president of the AANA in 1969–70. She graduated with a BS degree in Education from Fitchburg State College in Fitchburg, Massachusetts, which was affiliated with Burbank Hospital Collegiate Nurse Program. She received her anesthesia education from the Carney Hospital School of Anesthesia in Boston, later serving as the school's director.

1983   Goldie D. Brangman

Miss Brangman was AANA president in 1973–74. She served for many years as director of the Harlem Hospital Center School of Anesthesia for Nurses in New York, where she also held the positions of director of Continuing Education for the departments of anesthesia and respiratory therapy. Miss Brangman held certification as a respiratory therapist, physician's assistant, and medical illustrator. She earned a master's degree in education and business administration from City University of New York. Her many published works include *Medical Aspects of Drug Abuse* (Harper and Row), which she coauthored.

1984   Leah Evans Katz

Dr. Katz founded and served as director of the Master of Science program in Nurse Anesthesia at UCLA School of Medicine in Los Angeles. She earned a Doctor of Education degree in institutional management from Pepperdine School of Law in Los Angeles, staying on as adjunct associate professor. She was actively involved with the Council of Accreditation of Nurse Anesthesia Programs/Schools, serving as a senior on-site visitor and as an educational consultant. She was also a member of the Task Force on the Certification Examination with the Council on Certification of Nurse Anesthetists, and chairman of the Research Division of the AANA Education and Research Foundation. She has been a visiting professor at a number of schools and universities, and is a widely known lecturer on anesthesia and education.

1985   Celestine Harrigan

Some of Dr. Harrigan's most notable contributions to the nurse anesthesia profession occurred during her tenure as chairman of the Council on Accreditation of Nurse Anesthesia Programs/Schools. She was instrumental in developing and revising the Educational Standards and Guidelines for Nurse Anesthetists, and in helping to improve the accreditation process in general. She represented the Council before the US Office of Education of the Department of Health, Education and Welfare, which led to the Council's recognition by that office. She was also active as an on-site visitor and educational consultant for the Council on Accreditation. Dr. Harrigan earned her master's and doctoral degrees in physiology from Wayne State University. She later served as both assistant director of the Wayne State Nurse Anesthesia Program and as faculty member at the Wayne State University College of Pharmacy and Allied Health.

1986   Hershal Bradshaw (posthumously)

A well-known and respected nurse anesthesia educator, Mr. Bradshaw was lauded with the Helen Lamb Award posthumously. He was entering his second year as AANA director of Region 7 when he died in 1985. He founded and served as director of the University of

Texas Nurse Anesthesia Program in Houston, developing it into a master's degree program in 1982. Mr. Bradshaw had a distinguished military career, serving in the US Army for twenty years and holding the position of director of the Phase II Nurse Anesthesia Course at William Beaumont Army Medical Center in El Paso, Texas. His involvement and dedication to nurse anesthesia education were also evident in his four years of service as chairman of the AANA Education Committee, his service on the Council on Accreditation of Nurse Anesthesia Educational Programs/Schools, and his chairmanship of the Education Section of the AANA Education and Research Foundation. He was one of five editors of the book *Principles of Nurse Anesthesia Practice* (Appleton & Lange).

1987   Mary Alice Costello

For twenty-seven years Miss Costello served as director of the Cincinnati General Hospital School of Nurse Anesthesia, which she founded in 1945. She was one of the first nurse anesthetists to become adept in the administration of regional anesthesia, and became widely known for this skill, instructing nurse anesthetists from around the country. Miss Costello was also said to be the first nurse anesthetist to use a ventilator in the anesthetic care of a patient. In 1963–64, she was AANA president. Also during the 1960s, she joined a health-care team in Algeria, sponsored by CARE, serving as its sole anesthetist.

1988   Pauline Barbin

Ms. Barbin began her nurse anesthesia educator career in 1965 at Eastern Maine Medical Center, School of Nurse Anesthesia in Bangor, Maine, where she became a clinical and didactic instructor at the state's first school of nurse anesthesia. After she became director of the program in 1973, she restructured it into a twenty-four-month course. Ms. Barbin received her initial anesthesia education at Carney Hospital School of Anesthesia in Boston. She earned a bachelor of science at Thomas College in Waterville, Maine, and a master of education at the University of Maine at Orono in 1983. Ms. Barbin has held many offices and chairmanships within the Maine Association of Nurse Anesthetists.

Appendix VI

State Associations of Nurse Anesthesia by Year of Their Formation

Alabama	December 19, 1931
Minnesota	January 29, 1935
Ohio	April 4, 1935
California	May 7, 1935
Missouri	May 7, 1935
Pennsylvania	May 10, 1935
New York	May 23, 1935
Virginia	November 16, 1935
Texas	December 11, 1935
Oregon	December 30, 1935
Florida	February 8, 1936
Tennessee	February 13, 1936
Mississippi	May 4, 1936
Nebraska	September 5, 1936
Wisconsin	April 12, 1937
Indiana	April 14, 1937
Oklahoma	August 24, 1937
Michigan	December 29, 1937
Colorado	April 9, 1938
Georgia	August 13, 1938
Illinois	February 1, 1939
Washington	February 20, 1939
New Jersey	December 27, 1939
Louisiana	February 12, 1940
Arkansas	April 25, 1940
Massachusetts	July 11, 1940
Kansas	October 16, 1940
Iowa	December 3, 1940
North Carolina	May 10, 1941
Utah	November 5, 1941
Maryland	October 4, 1946

North Dakota	May 8, 1949
Connecticut	August 28, 1949
South Dakota	April 15, 1950
South Carolina	September 14, 1951
Montana	June 28, 1952
West Virginia	September 2, 1952
Delaware	March 12, 1953
Kentucky	February 18, 1956
Hawaii	March 17, 1956
Arizona	April 6, 1956
District of Columbia	April 20, 1956
Maine	May 10, 1956
Rhode Island	July 23, 1956
Idaho	August 4, 1956
New Hampshire	August 9, 1956
New Mexico	August 18, 1956
Nevada	August 23, 1956
Vermont	November 29, 1956
Wyoming	June 7, 1958
Alaska	June 17, 1960
Puerto Rico	April 14, 1962

Bibliographic Note

For general background in the history of health care in the United States, see Paul Starr, *The Social Transformation of American Medicine* (New York, 1982); Rosemary Stevens, *American Medicine and the Public Interest* (New Haven, 1971); Joseph F. Kett, *The Formation of the American Medical Profession: The Role of Institutions, 1780–1860* (New Haven, 1968), and William G. Rothstein, *American Physicians in the Nineteenth Century: From Sects to Science* (Baltimore and London, 1972). The work of Richard Harrison Shryock is always a pleasure to read; for example, *Medicine in America: Historical Essays* (Baltimore, 1966), *The Development of Modern Medicine: An Interpretation of the Social and Scientific Factors Involved* (New York, 1947), and "Nursing Emerges as a Profession: The American Experience," *Clio Medica* (1968), 3:131–147.

Thomas E. Keys, *The History of Surgical Anesthesia* (revised edition, New York, 1963) remains a classic on the subject, though it, like virtually all studies in the field, ignores the contributions of nurse anesthetists. A recent essay, beautifully written and unique in its inclusion of nurse anesthetists, is that of Roderick K. Calverley, M.D., "Anesthesia as a Specialty: Past, Present, and Future," in *Clinical Anesthesia,* ed. P. G. Barash, B. F. Cullen, and R. K. Stoelting (Philadelphia, 1989). The anesthesia centennial issue of *The Journal of the History of Medicine and Allied Sciences* (October, 1946), Vol. 1, No. 4, is a valuable source and the scholarly basis for much of Victor Robinson's popular *Victory Over Pain, A History of Anesthesia* (New York, 1946). Martin S. Pernick's *A Calculus of Suffering: Pain, Professionalism, and Anesthesia in Nineteenth-Century America* (New York, 1985) is an entertaining study with occasionally questionable conclusions, and contains a thorough bibliography. For a history of anesthesia as a physician specialty, see *The Genesis of Contemporary Anesthesiology,* ed. Perry P. Volpitto, M.D., and Leroy D. Vandam, M.D. (Springfield, IL, 1982). See also D. C. Lortie, "Doctors Without Patients: The Anesthesiologist—A New Medical Specialty" (master's thesis, University of Chicago, 1949). The Anesthesia History Association publishes a quarterly *Newsletter,* and can be reached through its editor, C. Ronald Stephen, M.D., 15801 Harris Ridge Court, Chesterfield, MO 63017.

Two recent and important studies of nursing history are those by Barbara Melosh and Susan M. Reverby. In *"The Physician's Hand," Work, Culture, and Conflict in American Nursing* (Philadelphia, 1982), Melosh considers the ways in which gender informs work, and, in particular, the medical division of labor mirrors the larger society. See also her essays "More than 'The Physician's Hand': Skill and Authority in Twentieth-Century Nursing," in *Women and Health in America, Historical Readings,* ed. Judith Walzer Leavitt (Madison, 1984), and "Every Woman is a Nurse: Work and Gender in the Emergence of Nursing," in *"Send Us a Lady Physician," Women Doctors in America, 1835–1920* (New York and London, 1985). Reverby's *Ordered to Care: The Dilemma of American Nursing, 1850–1945* (Cambridge and New York, 1987) provides a study of the political history of the hospital from the viewpoint of the nurse. Though neither work discusses nurse anesthetists, both help to illuminate the nurse anesthetist experience. An excellent bibliographic review-essay on the state of nursing history is that by Janet Wilson James, "Writing and Rewriting Nursing History," *The Bulletin of the History of Medicine* (1984), 58:568–584. A quarterly *Bulletin* is published by the American Association for the History of Nursing; its headquarters can be reached through Box 90803, Washington, DC 20090-0803.

The major resource for early nurse anesthetist history is Virginia S. Thatcher's, *History of Anesthesia, with Emphasis on the Nurse Specialist,* first published in 1953, reissued in 1984. For a recent study of the history of physician–nurse competition in anesthesia, see Ruth Vanderlaan Armstrong's dissertation, "Strategies for Staking Out Occupational Turf, an Analysis of Clinical Dietetics and Nurse Anesthesia in the Health Care Marketplace" (University of Illinois, Chicago, 1985); also, that of Doris Altemus Stoll, CRNA, "The Emerging Role of the Nurse Anesthetist in Medical Practice" (Northwestern University, 1988). Other aspects of the nurse anesthetist profession are treated in Mary Jeanette Mannino, CRNA, *The Nurse Anesthetist and the Law* (New York, 1982), and "From Nurse to Nurse Anesthetist: Effects of Professional Socialization on Career Development," a dissertation by Wynne Ryser Waugaman, CRNA (University of Pittsburgh, 1981). The essays of Ira Gunn, CRNA, are important in providing philosophic and historic contexts for understanding nurse anesthetist issues. See, for example, her "Current Nursing Issues and Their Implications for the Preparation of Nurse Anesthetists," *JAANA* (December, 1968), "Preparing Today's Nurse Anesthetists to Meet Contemporary Needs: A Philosophic and Pragmatic Approach," *JAANA* (February, 1974), and "Nurse Anesthetist–Anesthesiologist Relationships: Past, Present, and Implications for the Future," *JAANA* (April, 1975).

The British nurse in anesthesia is discussed by Daryl Pearce in her dissertation, "Specialization in Medicine: An Art or a Science? The Status of Anaesthetics" (The Wellcome Institute for the History of Medicine, 1988).

On the matter of recovering lost history, particularly that of women, see Gerda Lerner, *The Majority Finds Its Past: Placing Women in History* (New York and Oxford, 1979). Excellent studies of women in patriarchal society are Lerner's *The Creation of Patriarchy* (New York and Oxford, 1986) and Eva Figes, *Patriarchal Attitudes: Women in Society* (New York, 1987).

Notes

1. The Mother of Anesthesia

1. Virginia S. Thatcher, *History of Anesthesia, with Emphasis on the Nurse Specialist* (Philadelphia, 1953), 27–28.
2. Helen Clapesattle, *The Doctors Mayo* (Minneapolis, 1941), 427.
3. Related by Verne C. Hunt, MD, "The Present-Day Sphere of the Nurse Anesthetist," *Bulletin of the American Association of Nurse Anesthetists,* hereafter *BAANA,* Vol. 9, No. 4, November, 1941, 321.
4. Owen H. and Sarah D. Wangensteen, *The Rise of Surgery* (Minneapolis, 1978), 353.
5. Ibid.
6. Nicholas M. Greene, MD, "Anesthesia and the Development of Surgery (1846–96)," *Anesthesia and Analgesia,* Vol. 58, No. 1, Jan.–Feb., 1979, 11.
7. In William G. Rothstein, *American Physicians in the Nineteenth Century* (Baltimore and London, 1972), 257.
8. Ibid.
9. Rothstein, 258.
10. Greene, "Anesthesia and the Development of Surgery (1846–96)."
11. See, for example, Christopher Kauffman's two-volume history of the Alexian Brothers, *Tamers of Death* (New York, 1976) and *The Ministry of Healing* (New York, 1978).
12. Paul Starr, *The Social Transformation of American Medicine* (New York, 1982), 155.
13. In Ellen Davidson Baer, "The Conflictive Social Ideology of American Nursing: 1893, A Microcosm," unpublished PhD dissertation (New York University, 1982), 81–82.
14. Ibid.
15. Starr, 155.
16. Richard Shyrock, *The Development of Modern Medicine* (New York, 1947), 346–347.
17. Baer, 19.
18. "Medical Societies," New York Academy of Medicine, Condensed from Phonographic Reports for the Medical and Surgical Reporter, *Hospital Practice,* Vol. 3, No. 14, December 31, 1859, 305. D. H. Galloway, MD, "The Anesthetizer as a Specialist," *The Philadelphia Medical Journal,* May 27, 1899, 1175.
19. Henry J. Bigelow, "A History of the Discovery of Modern Anaesthesia," in *A Century of American Medicine.*
20. "Medical Societies."
21. "The Professional Anaesthetizer," Editorial, *Medical Record,* April 10, 1897, 522.
22. Saling Simon, MD, "The Relation of the Operator to the Anesthetist," *Medical Record,* February 12, 1898, 230.
23. Galloway, 1173.
24. Ibid. 1175.
25. Ibid.
26. Quoted in *Medical Review of Reviews,* ed. Boldt, 1897, 177.
27. Agatha C. Hodgins, "The Educational Objectives of the American Asso-

ciation of Nurse Anesthetists," *BAANA*, Vol. 9, No. 3, August, 1941, 164. A published report of a London-trained nurse anesthetist, Louise McMurray, being appointed to the staff of Salem Hospital, Salem, Massachusetts, in 1877, is the result of a misreading of the article's source, *From Charter to the Lookout: The Salem Hospital–A Brief History*, Walter G. Phippen, MD (Salem, Massachusetts, 1966). It seems McMurray joined that hospital some time between 1903 and 1917. I am very grateful to Dr. David J. Wilkinson, Dr. J. Alfred Lee, and Richard G. Ouellette, CRNA, for helping to correct the error in "Salem Hospital: Pioneer Quality Medical Care," *The Salem, Mass. Evening News*, August 12, 1987.

28. Mary Ewens, OP, "The Role of the Nun in Nineteenth-Century America: Variations on the International Theme," unpublished PhD dissertation (University of Minnesota, 1971).

29. Thatcher, 55.

30. Isabel Adams Hampton Robb, *Nursing: Its Principles and Practice for Hospital and Private Use* (New York, 1893).

31. Thatcher, 54, 95–96; "Award of Appreciation to Hospital Sisters Third Order of St. Francis," *AANA News Bulletin*, Vol. 8, No. 3, July, 1954, 1, 8.

32. Thatcher, 63–64.

33. Ibid., 54–55.

34. Ibid., 55.

35. Wilhelmina Gulotta, "Forty-four Years in Anesthesia," *BAANA*, Vol. 9, No. 4, November, 1941, 353–354.

36. Lawrence W. Littig, MD, "Anesthesia Fatalities in Iowa," *Tr. West. Surg. Gynec. Soc.*, 17:133, 1907, cited in Thatcher, 61.

37. *The Story of the First Fifty Years of the Mount Sinai Hospital, 1852–1902* (New York, 1944), 79; cited in Thatcher, 49.

38. James E. Moore, MD, in a discussion following presentation of Alice Magaw's "Observations Drawn from an Experience of Eleven Thousand Anesthesias," *Transactions of the Minnesota State Medical Association*, Thirty-Sixth Annual Meeting, 1904, 99. See also Littig, cited in Thatcher, 59.

39. Alice Magaw, "Observations in Anaesthesia," *Northwestern Lancet*, Vol. 19, 207–208.

40. George W. Crile, MD, *George Crile, An Autobiography*, Edited, with Sidelights, by Grace Crile, 2 Vol. (Philadelphia and New York, 1947), I, 168.

41. Clapesattle, 429.

42. Ibid., 427.

43. "The First Nurse Anesthetist," *Bulletin of the National Association of Nurse Anesthetists*, hereafter *BNANA*, Vol. 7, No. 2, May, 1939, 63.

44. Gerda Lerner, *The Majority Finds Its Past, Placing Women in History* (New York and Oxford, 1979).

45. The Magaw bibliography is: "Observations in Anesthesia," *Northwestern Lancet*, Vol. 19, May 15, 1899, 207–210; "Observations on 1092 Cases of Anesthesia from Jan. 1, 1899 to Jan. 1, 1900," *The St. Paul Medical Journal*, Vol. 2, January to December, 1900, 306–311; "A Report of 245 Cases of Anesthesia by Nitrous Oxide Gas and Ether," *The St. Paul*

Medical Journal, Vol. 3, No. 4, April, 1901, 231–233; "Observations Drawn from an Experience of Eleven Thousand Anesthesias," *Transactions of the Minnesota State Medical Association,* 1904, 91–99, with "Discussion" following, 99–102; "A Review of Over Fourteen Thousand Surgical Anesthesias," *Surgery, Gynecology and Obstetrics,* Vol. 3, December, 1906, 795–799.

46. Thatcher, 59.
47. Magaw, "A Review of Over Fourteen Thousand Surgical Anesthesias," reprinted in *BNANA,* Vol. 7, No. 2, May, 1939, 63.
48. Ibid., 64.
49. Ibid., 66.
50. Ibid., 68.
51. Ibid., 66.
52. Ibid., 64. For an interesting history of the use of hypnotism, see "Mesmerism and Surgery," George Rosen, *Journal of the History of Medicine and Allied Sciences,* October, 1946, 527–550. A contemporary study of therapeutic suggestion is "Improved Recovery and Reduced Postoperative Stay After Therapeutic Suggestions During General Anesthesia," Carlton Evans and P. H. Richardson, *The Lancet,* August 27, 1988, 491–493.
53. Charles H. Mayo, MD, in "Discussion" following Magaw, "Observations Drawn from an Experience of Eleven Thousand Anesthesias," 100–101.
54. Roderick K. Calverley, MD, "A Magnificent Heritage: The History of Pediatric Anesthesia," in *Anesthetic Management of Difficult and Routine Pediatric Patients,* ed. Frederic A. Berry, MD (New York, 1986), 7.
55. Littig, in Thatcher, 61.
56. J. M. Baldy, MD, "The Nurse as Anesthetist," *American Journal of Obstetrics,* Vol. 59, 1909, 997, cited in Thatcher, 81–82.
57. See Thatcher, 68–69.
58. Frances M. Dickinson-Berry, "Notes on the Administration of Anaesthetics in America, with Special Reference to the Practice at the Mayo Clinic," *Proceedings of the Royal Society of Medicine,* Vol. 6, Pt. 1, 1912–13, Section on Anaesthetics, December 6, 1912, 13–26. Mrs. Dickinson-Berry was the first woman member of Britain's Society of Anaesthetists, the first anesthesia society in the world. She became a member in 1894, one year after its founding. See Dr. Elizabeth P. Gibbs, "Three Lady Anaesthetists of 1893," scheduled for publication in the *Journal of the History of Anaesthesia Society,* I am grateful to its Editor, Dr. David J. Wilkinson, for a prepublication copy.
59. Dickinson-Berry, 15–16.
60. Ibid., 17.
61. H. J. Patterson, in "Discussion" following Dickinson-Berry, ibid., 25.
62. Dickinson-Berry, 20.
63. Magaw, "Observations on 1092 Cases of Anesthesia from Jan. 1, 1899 to Jan. 1, 1900," 309.
64. J. Blumfeld, MD, in "Discussion" following Dickinson-Berry, 21.
65. Fleming, ibid.
66. Patterson, ibid., 24.

67. Bellamy Gardner, ibid., 22.
68. Nicholas M. Greene, MD, *Anesthesiology and the University* (Philadelphia and Toronto, 1975), 16–17. See also his "A Consideration of Factors in the Discovery of Anesthesia and Their Effects on Its Development," *Anesthesiology*, Vol. 35, No. 5, November, 1971, 515–522.
69. Martin S. Pernick, *A Calculus of Suffering, Pain, Professionalism, and Anesthesia in Nineteenth-Century America* (New York, 1985), 88.

2. Up Against That Sort of Thing

1. Crile, "Greetings," *BNANA*, Vol. 4, No. 4, November, 1936, 183.
2. Crile, *George Crile, An Autobiography*, I, 194.
3. Crile, "Greetings," 182.
4. Ibid.
5. Cited in Thatcher, 73.
6. Crile, "Greetings," 183.
7. Crile, *George Crile, An Autobiography*, I, 195.
8. Crile, "Greetings," 183.
9. Ibid.
10. Crile, *George Crile, An Autobiography*, I, 195.
11. Miriam G. Shupp, in Thatcher, 73–74.
12. Crile, *George Crile, An Autobiography*, I, 196.
13. Ibid.
14. Ibid., 199.
15. Ibid., 198.
16. Ibid., 199.
17. Ibid.
18. Hodgins, "The Educational Objectives of the American Association of Nurse Anesthetists," 164–165.
19. Lucy E. Richards, *Journal of the American Association of Nurse Anesthetists*, hereafter, *JAANA*, Vol. 16, No. 4, November, 1948, 333.
20. Crile, *George Crile, An Autobiography*, I, 195.
21. Hodgins, "The Educational Objectives of the American Association of Nurse Anesthetists," 164.
22. Thatcher, 95.
23. Ibid.
24. Ibid., 96.
25. Crile, *George Crile, An Autobiography*, I, 199.
26. Hodgins, "The Educational Objectives of the American Association of Nurse Anesthetists," 165.
27. Crile, "Surgical Researches During the World War," *The Southern Medical Journal*, Vol. 13, No. 4, April, 1920, 267–271.
28. Ibid.
29. Arthur E. Guedel, MD, cited in Frederick W. Courington, MD and Roderick K. Calverley, MD, "Anesthesia on the Western Front: The Anglo-American Experience of World War I," *Anesthesiology*, Vol. 65, No. 6, December, 1986, 649.
30. Crile, quoted in Courington and Calverley, ibid.
31. Thatcher, 97.

32. Courington and Calverley, 649.
33. Mary J. Roche-Stevenson, "Front Line Anesthesia," *BAANA*, Vol. 10, No. 2, May, 1942, 72–73.
34. Ibid., 73.
35. Sophie Gran Winton, CRNA, unpublished interview with Marianne Bankert, June, 1986, AANA Archives.
36. Winton, quoted in Gustaf W. Olson, "The Nurse Anesthetist: Past, Present and Future," *BAANA*, Vol. 8, No. 4, November, 1940, 298.
37. Winton, "The War Years," *AANA News Bulletin*, Vol. 38, No. 11, 6.
38. Anne Penland, quoted from her Diary in Eleanor Lee, *History of the School of Nursing of the Presbyterian Hospital, New York, 1892–1942* (New York, 1942), 106–107. I am grateful to Dr. Roderick K. Calverley for this reference.
39. Cited in Thatcher, 100.
40. Crile, "Greetings," 184.
41. Daryl Pearce, "Specialization in Medicine: An Art or a Science? The Status of Anaesthetics," unpublished dissertation (The Wellcome Institute for the History of Medicine, 1988), 41. I am indebted to Dr. Christopher Lawrence for bringing this study to my attention.
42. Ibid., 42.
43. Ibid., 41.
44. Robert Emmett Farr, MD, in "Discussion" following Ralph M. Waters, MD, "Why the Professional Anesthetist," *The Journal-Lancet*, January 15, 1919, reprinted in *Selected Scientific Papers and Addresses of Ralph M. Waters, M.D.* (Cleveland, 1957), n.p.
45. Frederic W. Hewitt, MD, "The Past, Present, and Future of Anaesthesia" (1896).
46. Thatcher, 53.
47. See Ruth Vanderlaan Armstrong, "Strategies for Staking Out Occupational Turf, An Analysis of Clinical Dietetics and Nurse Anesthesia in the Health Care Marketplace," unpublished PhD dissertation (University of Illinois, Chicago, 1985).
48. Olson, 297.
49. Ibid., 297–298.
50. Crile, "Greetings," 182.
51. Ibid., 183.
52. Philemon E. Truesdale, cited in Thatcher, 111, who notes that Alice Hunt was then Truesdale's anesthetist.
53. Morton J. Tendler, MD, "Spinal Anesthesia and the Nurse Anesthetist," *BNANA*, Vol. 7, No. 3, August, 1939, 142–143.
54. Hewitt.
55. Thatcher, 88.
56. Albert J. Ochsner, MD, cited in Selma H. Calmes, MD, "The Surprising History of Women in Anesthesiology," presented at the annual meeting of the American Society of Anesthesiologists, October 16, 1984, unpublished paper, n.p.
57. Arthur Dean Bevan, MD, cited in Calmes, ibid.
58. Cited in Thatcher, 76.

59. See Calmes, "American Anesthesia from 1920 to 1950: Was It 'Women's Work?'" presented at the annual meeting of the American Association for the History of Medicine, May 5, 1984, unpublished paper.

60. Eleanor Seymour, MD, "The Present Status of Anesthesiology and the Anesthetist," *California State Journal of Medicine,* Vol. 18, October, 1920, 355.

61. The incident was reported by Frank McMechan in his "Anesthetic Supplement" of the *American Journal of Surgery,* October, 1921; cited by Thatcher, 117.

62. Lester C. Mark, MD, Leonard Brand, MD, and Richard J. Kitz, MD, "Emmanual M. Papper," in *The Genesis of Contemporary Anesthesiology,* ed. Perry P. Volpitto, MD, and Leroy D. Vandam, MD (Springfield, Illinois, 1982), 162.

63. Calmes, "The Surprising History of Women in Anesthesiology."

64. Ibid.

65. Stuart C. Cullen, MD, "An Account of the History of the Journal *Anesthesiology,*" *Anesthesiology,* Vol. 25, No. 4, July–August, 1964, 416.

66. Rosemary Stevens, *American Medicine and the Public Interest* (New Haven and London, 1971), 240.

67. Stuart C. Cullen, MD, "Emery Rovenstine," in *The Genesis of Contemporary Anesthesiology,* 80.

68. Calmes, "The Surprising History of Women in Anesthesiology."

3. A Very Personal Property Right

1. Ralph M. Waters, MD, "The Development of Anesthesiology in the United States, Personal Observations 1913–1936," *Journal of the History of Medicine and Allied Sciences,* Vol. 1, No. 4; reprinted in *Selected Scientific Papers and Addresses of Ralph Milton Waters, M.D.,* n.p.

2. Waters, "Why the Professional Anesthetist," *The Journal-Lancet,* January 15, 1919, reprinted in *Selected Papers and Addresses of Ralph Milton Waters, M.D.,* n.p. According to Leroy D. Vandam, MD, this, Waters's first paper, was "probably inspired by conversation with McMechan." See Vandam's "Early American Anesthetists, The Origins of Professionalism in Anesthesia," *Anesthesiology,* Vol. 38, No. 3, March, 1973, 264–274.

3. Waters, "Why the Professional Anesthetist."

4. C. E. McCauley, MD, ibid.

5. Crile, "Greetings," 183.

6. Thomas H. Seldon, "Francis Hoeffer McMechan," *The Genesis of Contemporary Anesthesiology,* 6.

7. Ibid., 8.

8. Ibid., 9.

9. Ibid., 10.

10. Ibid., 13.

11. Ibid.

12. Waters, "The Development of Anesthesiology in the United States."

13. Ibid.

14. Seldon, 9.

15. Ibid., 10.
16. Ibid., 11–12.
17. Ibid., 13.
18. Ibid.
19. Francis H. McMechan, MD, Editorial, Anesthesia Supplement, *American Journal of Surgery,* Vol. 29, No. 10, October, 1915, 155.
20. McMechan, Editorial, Anesthesia Supplement, *American Journal of Surgery,* Vol. 29, No. 4, April, 1915, 88.
21. McMechan, Editorial, Anesthesia Supplement, *American Journal of Surgery,* Vol. 29, No. 7, July, 1915, 120.
22. Thatcher, 110.
23. Ibid., 111.
24. Ibid., 112.
25. Ibid.
26. Ibid., 113.
27. Ibid.
28. Ibid., 112.
29. Ibid., 115.
30. Ibid., 115–116.
31. Ibid., 117–118.
32. Waters, "The Development of Anesthesiology in the United States, Personal Observations, 1913–46," n.p.
33. Ibid.

4. A Matter for Felicitation

1. Adeline Curtis, unpublished speech, AANA Archives.
2. Hilda Salomon, CRNA, unpublished interview with Janet McMahon, CRNA, 1979, AANA Archives.
3. Hodgins titled an autobiographical memoir, "A Narrative of Endeavor," unpublished manuscript, AANA Archives.
4. Ira Gunn, CRNA, "Current Nursing Issues and Their Implications for the Preparation of Nurse Anesthetists," *BAANA,* Vol. 36, No. 4, December, 1968, 416.
5. Hodgins, "The Educational Objectives of the American Association of Nurse Anesthetists," 165.
6. Ibid., 167.
7. Ibid.
8. Ibid.
9. Hodgins, May 9, 1931 letter of invitation, in Thatcher, 184.
10. Cited in Thatcher, 184–185.
11. Gertrude Fife, CRNA, unpublished interview with Janet McMahon, CRNA, AANA Archives.
12. Miriam Shupp, CRNA, unpublished interview with Ruth Satterfield, CRNA, AANA Archives.
13. Hodgins letter to Marie Louis, February 15, 1932, in Thatcher, 192.
14. Hodgins letter to Susan C. Francis, November 16, 1931, ibid., 190.
15. Marie Louis letter to Hodgins, December 28, 1931, ibid., 191.

16. Hodgins letter to Marie Louis, February 15, 1932, ibid., 192.
17. Hodgins letter to Marie Louis, March 22, 1932, ibid., 193.
18. Hodgins letter to Alma Scott, March 22, 1932, ibid., 193.
19. Alma Scott letter to Hodgins, March 24, 1932, ibid., 194.
20. Hodgins letter to Alma Scott, March 28, 1932, ibid.
21. Jane Van DeVrede letter to Hodgins, April 5, 1932, ibid., 194.
22. Hodgins letter to Van DeVrede, April 7, 1932, ibid., 195.
23. Hodgins letter to Helen Lamb, April 8, 1932, ibid., 197.
24. Susan C. Francis letter to Hodgins, May 3, 1932, ibid., 195.
25. Gunn, "Current Nursing Issues and Their Implications for the Preparation of Nurse Anesthetists," 416.
26. Hodgins, in Thatcher, 198.
27. Thatcher, 200–201.
28. Fife, unpublished interview.
29. John R. Mannix letter to Bert W. Caldwell, MD, May, 1933, in Thatcher, 201.
30. Caldwell letter to Fife, May 10, 1933, in Thatcher, 201.
31. Ibid., 201–202.
32. Shupp, unpublished interview.
33. Thatcher, 204.
34. Fife, unpublished interview.
35. Fife, "Report of the First Annual Meeting of the National Association of Nurse Anesthetists," *BNANA*, Vol. 1, No. 1, 1933, 43.
36. Evarts Graham, MD, "Letter of Greeting," ibid., 9.
37. Caldwell, "The Value of the Nurse Anesthetist to Present-Day Hospitalization," ibid., 14.
38. Ibid.
39. Hodgins, "President's Address," ibid., 10.
40. Ibid., 13.
41. Fife, "The Future of the Nurse Anesthetist," ibid., 16.
42. Ibid., 118–119.

5. Worlds at War

1. J. C. Doane, MD, "What the Hospital Anesthetist Should Be and Should Not Be," *BNANA*, Vol. 6, No. 1, February, 1938, 8.
2. Starr, 223.
3. Henry Hedden, MD, "The Place of the Nurse Anesthetist," *BNANA*, Vol. 6, No. 2, May, 1938, 60.
4. "Nurses as Anesthetists," Editorial, *American Journal of Surgery*, Vol. 28, No. 8, August, 1914, 321–322.
5. McMechan, "The Future of Anesthesia and Analgesia," Editorial, Anesthesia Supplement, *American Journal of Surgery*, Vol. 29, No. 4, April, 1915, 88.
6. McMechan, "The American College of Surgeons and Unlicensed Anesthetists," Editorial, ibid., Vol. 29, No. 7, July, 1915, 121.
7. Seldon, 12.
8. Hodgins, in Thatcher, 118.

9. *AANA News Bulletin,* November, 1984, 5–7.
10. Cited in Thatcher, 132–133.
11. Benjamin W. Black, MD, letter to Verne Hunt, MD, October 30, 1933, ibid., 141–142.
12. Ibid., 142.
13. Curtis, unpublished speech, AANA Archives. I have been unable to find corroborative evidence of her account of a 1932 affiliation between nurse anesthetists and the "National" Hospital Association.
14. "History and Progress of the California State Association of Nurse Anesthetists," unpublished manuscript, AANA Archives.
15. Curtis, in Thatcher, 133–135.
16. U. S. Webb letter to C. B. Pinkham, September 26, 1933, ibid., 136.
17. Ibid.
18. Ibid., 138.
19. Ibid.
20. Ibid., 138–139.
21. Ibid., 139.
22. Curtis, unpublished speech, AANA Archives.
23. Hunt letter to Black, October 27, 1933, in Thatcher, 141.
24. Kenneth E. Grant letter to Hunt, December 14, 1933, ibid., 142.
25. John G. Mott letter to Harry H. Wilson, April 19, 1934, ibid., 143.
26. Retraction sent to Mott, ibid., 144.
27. Reporter's transcript on appeal, Vol. 1, 1–3, ibid., 145.
28. Thatcher, 145.
29. Ibid., 146.
30. Ibid.
31. Ibid., 147.
32. Ibid., 148.
33. Board of Trustees proceedings, *The Bulletin of the Los Angeles County Medical Association,* Vol. 66, 699, 1936, in Thatcher, 149.
34. W. Chalmers-Francis, Letter to the Editors, *Medical Economics,* January, 1937.
35. Hunt, "The Present-Day Sphere of the Nurse Anesthetist," 322.
36. Hunt letter to Helen Lamb, October, 1941, AANA Archives.
37. Lamb letter to Hunt, October, 1941, AANA Archives.
38. Anne M. Campbell, "Report of the Executive Secretary," *BAANA,* Vol. 12, No. 4, November, 1944, 238.
39. Hodgins letter to Curtis, June 20, 1932, AANA Archives.
40. Hodgins letter to Marie Louis, February 15, 1932, in Thatcher, 192.
41. Hodgins letter to Curtis, June 20, 1932.
42. Fife, "The Future of the Nurse Anesthetist," *BNANA,* Vol. 1, No. 1, 1933, 18–19.
43. Fife, "Organization of the American Association of Nurse Anesthetists," unpublished memoir, 1971, AANA Archives.
44. Ibid.
45. Fife, unpublished interview with Janet McMahon, CRNA, AANA Archives.
46. Fife, in Thatcher, 210–211.

47. Fife, unpublished interview
48. Hodgins letter to Fife, August 23, 1934, in Thatcher, 212.
49. Fife letter to Hodgins, August 29, 1934, ibid.
50. Hodgins letter to Fife, September 15, 1934, ibid., 212–213.
51. "Revised report of the Educational Committee: Recommendations Regarding Schools of Anesthesia for Nurses," *BNANA*, Vol. 5, No. 2, May, 1937, 310.
52. Fife, letter to Board of Trustees of NANA, September 30, 1935, in Thatcher, 224.
53. Ibid.
54. "Report of Education Committee," *BNANA*, Vol. 4, No. 4, November, 1936, 191.
55. Ibid., 190.
56. "Report of the Education Committee," *BNANA*, Vol. 5, No. 4, November, 1937, 414.
57. Frederick P. Haugen, MD, "The American Board of Anesthesiology, Inc." in *The Genesis of Contemporary Anesthesiology*, 217.
58. Stevens, 241.
59. "Minutes of the Meeting of the Board of Trustees of the Nurse Anesthetist Association," November 26, 1938, AANA Archives.
60. Shupp, unpublished interview.
61. Fife, unpublished interview. Regretfully, my request to review the ABA documents discussed by Haugen and Stevens was denied (Alan D. Sessler, MD, Secretary-Treasurer, The American Board of Anesthesiology, letter to Marianne Bankert, August 23, 1988).
62. Hodgins, "Introducing the Department of Education," *BAANA*, Vol. 8, No. 2, May, 1940, 102–103.
63. Ibid., 103.
64. Hodgins letter to Lamb, July 12, 1940, AANA Archives.
65. Beatrice M. Quin, RN, "Anesthesia in Army Hospitals," *BAANA*, Vol. 8, No. 4, November, 1940, 281–282.
66. Ibid., 282.
67. "Report of the Committee on Education," *BAANA*, Vol. 11, No. 4, November, 1943, 259.
68. Shupp, "The Progress of the Nurse Anesthetist," *BAANA*, Vol. 9, No. 2, May, 1941, 101.
69. Letter from Major Julia O. Flikke, in unsigned Editorial, "Present Status of Nurse Anesthetists in the United States Army and Navy, *BAANA*, Vol. 9, No. 3, August, 1941, 232.
70. Letter from US Navy Rear Admiral Ross T. McIntire, ibid.
71. Ibid.
72. Gertrude Fife, Editorial, *BAANA*, Vol. 10, No. 1, February, 1942, 42.
73. Unsigned Editorial, "Current Status of the Nurse Anesthetist Entering Military Service," *BAANA*, Vol. 10, No. 2, May, 1942, 125.
74. Ibid.
75. For a discussion of the recognition of medical specialists by the military, see Stevens, 277–280.
76. Lieutenant Colonel Katherine E. Baltz, "The Value of Special Training

in Anesthesia for the Army Nurse," *JAANA,* Vol. 15, No. 3, August, 1947, 139.

77. Unsigned Editorial, *BAANA,* Vol. 10, No. 3, August, 1942, 135.
78. Baltz, 138–139.
79. Edith A. Aynes, *From Nightingale to Eagle, An Army Nurse's History* (New Jersey, 1973), 89, 94–96.
80. Fife, unpublished interview.
81. Barbara M. Draper, CRNA, letter to Roderick K. Calverley, MD, January 18, 1988. I am grateful to both of them for sharing this with me.
82. Baltz, 140.
83. Ibid., 139.
84. Evelyn K. King, "Letters from Members," *BAANA,* Vol. 13, No. 4, November, 1945, 37–38.
85. "Navy Nurse Cited for Meritorious Service," *BAANA,* Vol. 13, No. 4, November, 1945, 42.
86. "Cited for War Service," *BAANA,* Vol. 14, No. 1, February, 1946.
87. Annie Mealer letter to Edith A. Aynes, in Aynes, 178–181.
88. Susan M. Hartmann, *American Women in the 1940s: The Home Front and Beyond* (Boston, 1982), 41.
89. Aynes, 257–258.
90. Ibid., 248–249.
91. "Anesthesia: A Career for the Graduate Nurse," Gertrude Fife anonymous author, *BAANA,* Vol. 10, No. 2, May, 1942, 103.
92. "Report of the Executive Secretary," *BAANA,* Vol. 10, No. 4, November, 1942, 243.
93. "Special Committee," *BAANA,* Vol. 10, No. 4, November, 1942, 259.
94. Rosalie McDonald, CRNA, "Report of the President," *BAANA,* Vol. 11, No. 4, November, 1943, 254–255.
95. "Committee on Education," *BAANA,* Vol. 12, No. 4, November, 1944, 254.
96. Lamb, "President's Report," *BAANA,* Vol. 10, No. 4, November, 1942, 240.
97. Anne M. Campbell, "Report from Headquarters," *BAANA,* Vol. 12, No. 2, May, 1944, 82.
98. Lamb, "President's Report," *BAANA,* Vol. 10, No. 4, November, 1942, 242; McDonald, "Report of the President," *BAANA,* Vol. 11, No. 4, November, 1943, 255.
99. Hodgins, "Editorial," *BAANA,* Vol. 13, No. 1, February, 1945, 32–33.
100. "In Memoriam: George W. Crile," Agatha Hodgins, Lou E. Adams, and Frank S. Gibson, MD, *BAANA,* Vol. 11, No. 1, February, 1943, 6–9.

6. Everything Is Under Control

1. Lucy E. Richards, "Report of the President," *JAANA,* Vol. 15, No. 4, November, 1947, 186.
2. Fife, unpublished interview.
3. Richards, "Florence A. McQuillen Appointed Executive Director," *JAANA,* Vol. 16, No. 1, February, 1948. 5.
4. Ibid.

5. "Who Should Give Anesthetics? Here's What Hospitals Think," *Hospital Management,* April, 1948.

6. Ibid.

7. "ACS Resolution on Nurse Anesthetists," *AANA News Bulletin,* Vol. 2, No. 1, March, 1948, 6.

8. "Resolution on Nurse Anesthetists," *JAANA,* Vol. 16, No. 1, February, 1948, 70.

9. AANA President Richards had requested action from the AMA in a letter to Dr. George Lull, Secretary, January 22, 1948 (*AANA News Bulletin,* Vol. 2, No. 1, March, 1948, 4). The AMA response, condemning the publicity, was reported in *JAANA,* Vol. 16, No. 1, May, 1948, 155.

10. Shupp, "The Answer is 'Yes,'" *JAANA,* Vol. 15, No. 3, August, 1947, 117–118.

11. Kenneth B. Babcock, MD, "The Hospital's Dilemma," *JAANA,* Vol. 18, No. 1, February, 1950, 35.

12. Ibid., 37.

13. "Anesthesia Costs Rise as Doctors Take Over," Walter Lerch, *Cleveland Plain Dealer,* June 21, 1950, AANA Archives, Notebook 1950–51.

14. Fife, "Is the Situation Serious?" *JAANA,* Vol. 15, No. 2, May, 1947, 65.

15. Richards, "AANA: Past, Present, and Future," *JAANA,* Vol. 16, No. 3, August, 1948, 174.

16. Richard G. Zepernick, Edwin G. Hyde, Mohammad Ali Naraghi, "John Adriani," in *The Genesis of Contemporary Anesthesiology,* 138–139.

17. Ibid., 139.

18. Albert M. Betcher, MD, "Historical Development of the American Society of Anesthesiologists, Inc.," ibid., 205.

19. Florence A. McQuillen, "Minutes of the Board of Directors of the AANA," 1948, AANA Archives.

20. Charles T. Dolezal, MD, "Accreditation–A Job for Voluntary Agencies," *AANA News Bulletin,* Vol. 4, No. 2, June, 1950, 6.

21. "Accreditation Advisors Appointed, Agreement for Two Year Study," *AANA News Bulletin,* Vol. 5, No. 2, April, 1951, 1.

22. Editorial, "The Goal of Accreditation," *JAANA,* Vol. 19, No. 2, May, 1951, 69. Dr. Cameron Meredith subsequently replaced Lowe.

23. Fife, "AANA 25th Anniversary," Editorial, *JAANA,* Vol. 24, No. 1, February, 1956, 4.

24. Verna Bean, "Open Letter to the Membership," *AANA News bulletin,* Vol. 5, No. 2, April, 1951, 2,4.

25. Bean served in England, Ireland, and France. In a radio interview (with Florence McQuillen) on September 23, 1947, for station WTMV, St. Louis, Missouri, she reflected on the use of pentothal, which was dubbed the "GI cocktail," and was administered to the wounded on a "cocktail date." AANA archives, unnumbered notebook.

26. "National Press Club Honors AANA Member," *AANA News Bulletin,* Vol. 7, No. 3, July, 1953, 1.

27. "Mollie Younger and the Big Story," *AANA News Bulletin,* Vol. 8, No. 4, October, 1954, 20.

28. Madeline McConnell, "The Director of Nursing Education," *JAANA*, Vol. 14, No. 2, May, 1946, 42.
29. Editorial, "Nursing Organization," *JAANA*, Vol. 16, No. 1, February, 1948.
30. Louise Knapp, "Strength through Cooperation," *JAANA*, Vol. 16, No. 1, February, 1948, 8.
31. Verna M. Rice, in "Nurse Anesthetists and the A.N.A.," *JAANA*, Vol. 19, No. 19, No. 2, May, 1951, 62–64.
32. Louise Schwarting, in "Nurse Anesthetists and the A.N.A.," ibid., 66.
33. Mildred G. Rumpf letter to McQuillen, November 20, 1951, AANA Archives.
34. Editorial, "The 1952 Biennial Convention," *JAANA*, Vol. 20, No. 3, August, 1952, 154.
35. Janet Geister, "We Must Walk Together," *JAANA*, Vol. 27, No. 2, May, 1959, 123.
36. Ibid., 120.
37. Gunn, "Current Nursing Issues and Their Implications for the Preparation of Nurse Anesthetists," *JAANA*, Vol. 35, No. 4, December, 1968, 416–417.
38. Gunn, "Preparing Today's Nurse Anesthetists to Meet Contemporary Needs: A Philosophic and Pragmatic Approach," *JAANA*, Vol. 42, No. 1, February, 1974, 33.
39. Salomon, "President's Report," *BNANA*, Vol. 4, No. 4, 186.
40. Shupp, unpublished interview.
41. Richard Redman, "The Nurse and the Draft in the Vietnam War," *Bulletin of the American Association for the History of Nursing*, Winter, 1986, No. 10.
42. Cindy Gurney, Major, ANC, "The Nurse and the Draft," ibid., Spring–Summer, 1986, No. 11.
43. John A. Jenicek, Colonel MC, Ret., "Viet Nam–New Challenge for the Army Nurse Anesthetist," *JAANA*, Vol. 35, No. 3, October, 1967, 349.
44. David R. Fletcher, CRNA, letter to Marianne Bankert, July 6, 1988, AANA Archives.
45. Patricia L. Walsh, CRNA, *Forever Sad the Hearts* (New York, 1982), 3, 51–52.
46. Jenicek, 348.
47. Betcher, MD, 200.
48. Ibid., 201.
49. Statistics gathered from "Survey of Anesthesia Services: 1955," Jessie L. Compton, Marie N. Bader, Minnie V. Haas, and Agnes M. Lange, *JAANA*, Vol. 23, No. 4, November, 1955, 223–235; "Survey of Anesthesia Service: 1965, A Ten-Year Comparison," Carma E. Mahler, CRNA, Dolores E. Biggins, CRNA, and Jo Ann Kaiser, CRNA, *JAANA*, Vol. 33, No. 3, Ocotober, 1965, 298–308; "Survey of Anesthesia Service: 1971," Dolores E. Biggins, CRNA, Alice Bakutis, CRNA, Vella G. Nelson, CRNA, and Martha Petraitis, CRNA, *JAANA*, Vol. 39, No. 3, October, 1971, 371–379.
50. Betcher, 203.

51. Mary Alice Costello, CRNA, quoted in Betcher, 204–205.
52. Adriani letter to McQuillen, December 7, 1965, AANA Archives.
53. McQuillen, "Position Statement," in response to Adriani request of December 7, 1965, AANA Archives.
54. McQuillen, Memo to the AANA Board of Trustees, November 3, 1965.
55. "ASA-AANA Statement," *AANA News Bulletin*, Vol. 22, No. 1, January, 1968, 3.
56. "ASA-AANA Joint Committee Statement," *AANA News Bulletin*, Vol. 24, No. 4, July, 1970, 4–5.
57. "Joint Statement of the ASA and AANA Concerning Qualifications of Individuals Administering Anesthetics," *AANA News Bulletin*, Vol. 26, No. 1, 3.
58. Virginia A. Gaffey, CRNA, "Report of the President," *AANA News Bulletin*, Vol. 25, No. 6, 13.
59. Goldie D. Brangman, CRNA, unpublished interview with Janet McMahon, CRNA, AANA Archives.
60. Ibid.
61. Ibid.
62. McQuillen, "Report of the Executive Director," *AANA News Bulletin*, Vol. 25, No. 6, December, 1971, 4.
63. McQuillen, "Report of the Executive Director," ibid., Vol. 17, No. 4, November, 1963, 44.
64. Costello, unpublished interview with Janet McMahon, CRNA, AANA Archives.
65. Ibid.
66. John S. Lundy, MD, "From This Point in Time: Some Memories of My Part in the History of Anesthesia," *JAANA*, Vol. 34, No. 2, April, 1966, 100.
67. Costello, unpublished interview.
68. McQuillen, "Director Emeritus Report," *AANA News Bulletin*, Vol. 24, No. 6, November, 1970, 15–16.
69. McQuillen, "From the Plaza," *AANA News Bulletin*, Vol. 24, No. 2, March, 1970, 2.

7. A Return to Roots

1. Brangman, "President's Address," *AANA News Bulletin*, Vol. 28, No. 6, November, 1974, 8.
2. Starr, 379.
3. Gunn, "Chronological Outline Pertaining to the Nurse in Anesthesia within the United States, Particularly with Reference to Physician Support and Challenges," 1986, unpublished paper, AANA Archives, 7.
4. Gunn, quoted in Editorial, *JAANA*, Vol. 29, No. 2, April, 1975, 105.
5. Pearl Dunkley, ibid., 103–104.
6. Gunn, "Chronological Outline," 8.
7. "AANA Reaffirms Its Position on Credentialing: Views Formation of FNAS with Concern," *AANA News Bulletin*, Vol. 30, No. 1, January, 1976, 1, 36.

8. Betcher, 207.
9. Doris Altemus Stoll, CRNA, "The Emerging Role of the Nurse Anesthetist in Medical Practice," unpublished PhD dissertation (Northwestern University, 1988) 143. See also, Dolores E. Biggins, CRNA, tribute to Baum in "President's Message," *AANA News Bulletin*, Vol. 30, No. 3, May, 1976, 3.
10. *AANA News Bulletin*, Vol. 30, No. 1.
11. Z. Danilevicius, MD, *JAMA* Editorial, "Cooperation and Educational Efforts Lead to Better Service," reprinted in *JAANA*, Vol. 43, No. 3, June, 1975, 238–239, "*JAMA* Recognizes AANA and ASA Efforts in the Field of Anesthesiology."
12. Jeffrey A. Brown, MD, "Professional Autonomy and the Nurse Anesthetist," *AANA News Bulletin*, Vol. 30, No. 1, 1.
13. Barbara Melosh, *"The Physician's Hand": Work, Culture, and Conflict in American Nursing* (Philadelphia, 1982), 20.
14. Gunn, "Nurse Anesthetist-Anesthesiologist Relationships: Past, Present, and Implications for the Future," *JAANA*, Vol. 43, No. 2, April, 1975, 136.
15. Ibid., 137.
16. John W. Ditzler, MD, ASA President's Annual Report, quoted in Nancy Fevold, CRNA, "Cooperation, Communication, and Coexistence: Is It Attainable?" *AANA News Bulletin*, Vol. 30, No. 6, November, 1976, 2.
17. John F. Garde, CRNA, "Identity and Involvement," *JAANA*, Vol. 45, No. 4, August, 1977, 379.
18. See, for example, John Adriani, MD, letter to the editor, *ASA Newsletter*, September, 1984, 10.
19. Ronald F. Caulk, CRNA, letter to Marianne Bankert, November 3, 1988.
20. Ibid.
21. Sandra M. Maree, CRNA, and Judith A. Ryan, PhD, quoted in "Victory for CRNAs–Medicare Direct Reimbursement Implemented on January 1," *AANA News Bulletin*, Vol. 43, No. 2, February, 1989.
22. Gunn, "Chronological Outline," 10–11. I am grateful to Ira Gunn for her assistance in this discussion.
23. Ibid.
24. Gene A. Blumenreich, "The Irrelevant Issue of Surgeon's Liability," *JAANA*, Vol. 53, No. 5, October, 1985, 459.
25. Ibid.
26. Fifth Circuit Court of Appeals, cited by Blumenreich "The AANA's *amicus curiae* Brief," *JAANA*, Vol. 51, No. 4, August, 1983, 411. See also William R. Kucera, "The Courts Look at the Exclusive Contract for Providing Anesthesia Services," *JAANA*, Vol. 49, No. 2, April, 1981, 174–175.
27. Justice Sandra D. O'Connor, quoted in Blumenreich, "Jefferson Parish Hospital v. Hyde–The Last Chapter," *JAANA*, Vol. 52, No. 4, August, 1984.

Index of Names